"This book extends the ethics of Lacanian psychoanalysis in the clinic to the symbolic and real beyond the clinic. The position of the analyst in the world is crucial for our time, and this book gathers some of the wisest, clearest voices in our field."

– **Annie G. Rogers, PhD, psychoanalyst, Lacanian School of Psychoanalysis; Professor Emerita of Psychoanalysis and Clinical Psychology, Hampshire College**

"An extraordinary collection, which foregrounds and advances the radical progressive impulse that has arguably always been inherent in Lacanian clinical social theory. Moving from questions of political emancipation, capitalist *jouissance* and Lacan's Marx, to the pragmatic concerns of homelessness, immigrant identity, violence and community mental health – and, of course, the paramount concern of how we might effectively *decolonize Lacan* – this volume makes an invaluable contribution to how we might reframe and respond to the most pressing socio-political and ideological dilemmas of our times."

– **Derek Hook, PhD, author, *Six Moments in Lacan***

"These urgent and original essays by experienced clinicians and distinguished scholars reclaim the too often disavowed political power of the unconscious, thus freeing psychoanalysis as a tool for social change. This stellar collection is a work of emancipatory radicality that changes the way we think about and with psychoanalysis."

– **Patricia Gherovici, PhD, psychoanalyst; author, *Transgender Psychoanalysis: A Lacanian Perspective on Sexual Difference***

Psychoanalysis, Politics, Oppression and Resistance

This innovative text addresses the lack of literature regarding intersectional approaches to psychoanalysis, underscoring the importance of thinking through race, class, and gender within psychoanalytic theory and practice.

The book tackles the widespread perception of psychoanalysis today as a discipline detached from the progressive ideals of social responsibility, institutional psychotherapy, and community mental health. Bringing together a range of international contributions, the collection explores issues of class, politics, oppression, and resistance within the field of psychoanalysis in cultural, theoretical, and clinical contexts. It shows how, in contrast to this misperception, psychoanalysis has been attentive to these ideals from its origins, as well as demonstrating how it continues to be relevant today, through wide-ranging conceptual discussions of the anti-globalization, Black Lives Matter, and #MeToo movements.

Written in an accessible style, *Psychoanalysis, Politics, Oppression and Resistance* will be essential reading for practicing psychoanalysts as well as academics and students in a range of humanities and social sciences fields.

Chris Vanderwees, PhD, RP, is a psychoanalyst and registered psychotherapist at St. John the Compassionate in Toronto, Canada.

Kristen Hennessy, PhD, is a licensed psychologist and advanced certified trauma practitioner in Pennsylvania. Her work appears in the collection *Lacanian Psychoanalysis with Babies, Children, and Adolescents* (Routledge, 2017).

The Lines of the Symbolic in Psychoanalysis Series

Series Editor: Ian Parker

Manchester Psychoanalytic Matrix

Psychoanalytic clinical and theoretical work is always embedded in specific linguistic and cultural contexts and carries their traces, traces which this series attends to in its focus on multiple contradictory and antagonistic 'lines of the Symbolic'. This series takes its cue from Lacan's psychoanalytic work on three registers of human experience, the Symbolic, the Imaginary and the Real, and employs this distinctive understanding of cultural, communication and embodiment to link with other traditions of cultural, clinical and theoretical practice beyond the Lacanian symbolic universe. The Lines of the Symbolic in Psychoanalysis Series provides a reflexive reworking of theoretical and practical issues, translating psychoanalytic writing from different contexts, grounding that work in the specific histories and politics that provide the conditions of possibility for its descriptions and interventions to function. The series makes connections between different cultural and disciplinary sites in which psychoanalysis operates, questioning the idea that there could be one single correct reading and application of Lacan. Its authors trace their own path, their own line through the Symbolic, situating psychoanalysis in relation to debates which intersect with Lacanian work, explicating it, extending it and challenging it.

Toward a Feminist Lacanian Left
Psychoanalytic Theory and Intersectional Theory
Alicia Valdés

The Marx Through Lacan Vocabulary
A Compass for Libidinal and Political Economies
Christina Soto van der Plas, Edgar Miguel Juárez-Salazar, Carlos Gómez Camarena and David Pavón-Cuéllar

Psychoanalysis, Politics, Oppression and Resistance
Lacanian Perspectives
Chris Vanderwees and Kristen Hennessy

For more information about this series, please visit: www.routledge.com

Psychoanalysis, Politics, Oppression and Resistance

Lacanian Perspectives

Edited by Chris Vanderwees
and Kristen Hennessy

Routledge
Taylor & Francis Group
LONDON AND NEW YORK

Cover image: © Getty Images

First published 2022
by Routledge
4 Park Square, Milton Park, Abingdon, Oxon OX14 4RN

and by Routledge
605 Third Avenue, New York, NY 10158

Routledge is an imprint of the Taylor & Francis Group, an informa business

British Library Cataloguing-in-Publication Data
A catalogue record for this book is available from the British Library

Library of Congress Cataloging-in-Publication Data
A catalog record for this book has been requested

ISBN: 978-1-032-07913-4 (hbk)
ISBN: 978-1-032-07916-5 (pbk)
ISBN: 978-1-003-21207-2 (ebk)

DOI: 10.4324/9781003212072

Typeset in Bembo
by Apex CoVantage, LLC

Contents

Acknowledgements

The editors are especially grateful for Ian Parker's support of this book. We would also like to thank Ellie Duncan and Susannah Frearson at Routledge for their help during the publishing process. We would also like to thank the Lacan Toronto working group for the many opportunities for discussions and presentations on topics related to psychoanalysis. Many thanks to all of the contributors for these inspiring chapters.

An earlier version of Chapter 4 was published as Vanderwees, Chris. "Dwelling on the Direction of the Treatment for the Homeless Subject." *Psychoanalytische Perspectieven*. 38.4 (2020): 411–423. The revised version is printed in this present collection with permissions.

Chris Vanderwees is very thankful to MCL for all of her support. He is also especially grateful to JH for all of her kindness and encouragement.

Contributors

Daniel Adleman is Assistant Professor of Writing and Rhetoric at the University of Toronto. Holding a PhD in English Language and Literature from the University of British Columbia, he teaches and writes primarily about the myriad relationships between rhetoric, psychoanalysis, media studies, and social change. He has recently published essays in *The Canadian Review of American Studies*, *Canadian Literature Quarterly*, *Crossing Borders* (ARP, 2020), *Utopia and Dystopia in the Age of Trump* (Rowman & Littlefield, 2019), and *Performing Utopias in the Contemporary Americas* (Palgrave Macmillan, 2017). In 2012, he co-founded the Vancouver Institute of Social Research, an ongoing critical theory free school held at downtown Vancouver's Or Gallery.

Clint Burnham is Professor and Chair of the Graduate Program in English, Simon Fraser University, Vancouver, Canada. He was born in Comox, British Columbia, which is on the traditional territory of the K'ómoks (Sathloot) First Nation, centred historically on kwaniwsam. He lives and teaches on the traditional ancestral territories of the Coast Salish peoples, including traditional territories of the Squamish (Sḵwx̱wú7mesh Úxwumixw), Tsleil-Wauțuth (səl̓ilw̓ətaʔɬ), Musqueam (xʷməθkʷəy̓əm), and Kwikwetlem (kʷikʷəƛ̓əm) Nations. He is a founding member and president of the Vancouver Lacan Salon; his most recent books include *Fredric Jameson and the Wolf of Wall Street* (Bloomsbury, 2016) and *Does the Internet Have an Unconscious? Slavoj Žižek and Digital Culture* (Bloomsbury, 2018).

Sheila L. Cavanagh is a Professor of Sociology at York University and former Chair of the Canadian Sexuality Studies Association. She teaches and researches gender and sexuality studies with a focus on feminist, queer, cultural, and psychoanalytic theories. She is the author of *Sexing the Teacher: School Sex Scandals and Queer Pedagogies* (University of British Columbia Press, 2007) and *Queering Bathrooms: Gender, Sexuality, and the Hygienic Imagination* (University of Toronto Press, 2010) as well as the co-editor (with Angela Failler and Rachel Alpha Johnston Hurst) of *Skin,*

Culture and Psychoanalysis (Palgrave Macmillan, 2013) and the co-editor of a special double-issue of *Transgender Studies Quarterly*, "Transgender and Psychoanalysis" (2017).

Bo Earle is Assistant Professor of English at the University of British Columbia, Canada. He is the author of *Post-Personal Romanticism: Democratic Terror, Prosthetic Poetics, and the Comedy of Modern Ethical Life* (Ohio State University Press, 2017).

Kristen Hennessy is a licensed psychologist and advanced certified trauma practitioner in Pennsylvania. She provides trauma-informed psychoanalytic treatment of children and adolescents with histories of complex trauma, many of whom are or were in the foster care system. She collaborates with parents, foster parents, caseworkers, schools, and others in the service of continuity of care. Kristen also provides training to schools, foster care agencies, foster parents, biological parents, and others involved in the lives of children with complex trauma. Her work appears in the collection *Lacanian Psychoanalysis with Babies, Children, and Adolescents* (Routledge, 2017).

Christopher Meyer is an Analyst, Supervising Analyst and Faculty of the San Francisco Lacanian School of Psychoanalysis. He has a private practice in Los Angeles where he works with young adults, adults, couples, and families. He is the former Doctoral Program Director at The Maple Counseling Center where he continues to supervise interns. He is a member of GIFRIC, a member of the Freudian School of Québec, and a founding member of the California Circle of the Freudian School of Québec.

Debora Kirschbaum Nitkin is a psychoanalytic psychotherapist and a Lacanian psychoanalyst in private practice in Toronto, in addition to her position as retired faculty member at the Bloomberg Faculty of Nursing, University of Toronto. She was formerly an Associate Professor at the State University of Campinas in Brazil where she coordinated the "Nucleum of Research in Psychoanalysis, Nursing and Mental Health."

Ian Parker is a practising psychoanalyst in Manchester, Honorary Professor in Education at the University of Manchester, and Visiting Professor in Psychosocial Studies at Birkbeck, University of London. He is the author of *Lacanian Psychoanalysis: Revolutions in Subjectivity* (Routledge, 2011).

David Pavón-Cuéllar is Professor of Psychology at Universidad Michoacana de San Nicolás de Hidalgo in Morelia, Mexico. He has taught psychoanalysis at the University of Paris VIII.

Alireza Taheri provides psychoanalytic psychotherapy in private practice in Toronto, where he is also actively involved in teaching Lacanian theory at the Toronto Psychoanalytic Institute and Society. Alireza is a permanent faculty member of HamAva Psychoanalytic Institute in Tehran (Iran), where he teaches psychoanalytic theory and practice. He is also engaged in writing articles on philosophy and psychoanalysis and is presently the editor-in-chief and book review editor of *Psychoanalytic Discourse* (an independent international journal for the clinical, theoretical, and cultural discussion of psychoanalysis).

Chris Vanderwees is a psychoanalyst and registered psychotherapist at St. John the Compassionate in Toronto, Canada. He is a member of the Lacanian School of Psychoanalysis and an affiliate and research guest of the Toronto Psychoanalytic Society. He has previously received SSHRC Doctoral and Postdoctoral Fellowships for his research on trauma, language, and psychoanalysis. His articles and translations can be found in *American Imago*, the *International Journal of Psychoanalysis*, the *European Journal of Psychoanalysis*, the *Canadian Journal of Psychoanalysis*, and *Psychoanalytische Perspectieven*.

Eve Watson is a psychoanalytic practitioner, clinical supervisor, and academic. She is involved in teaching and training in psychoanalysis, psychotherapy, and teacher education and specializes in teaching sexuality studies at postgraduate and undergraduate levels. She is currently teaching in the areas of psychology and sociology in education; sexuality and the social world; and sexuality for psychotherapy training. Her book (with Dr. Noreen Giffney) is *Clinical Encounters in Sexuality: Psychoanalytic Practice and Queer Theory* (Punctum Books, 2017). She is widely published in Irish and international journals and conference proceedings and annually speaks at conferences and public events in Ireland, Europe, the USA, and Canada. She is currently the editor of *Lacunae: The APPI International Journal for Psychoanalysis*, a peer-reviewed journal.

Series Preface

What is politics but an attempt to symbolize the world? That attempt at symbolization takes place today in conditions of alienation and poverty for many and entitlement and power for a few, and it is usually from that few that the analysands who make use of psychoanalysis come into the clinic and from that few that the psychoanalysts themselves emerge as those who may then come to think of themselves as enlightened rather than privileged.

Some psychoanalysts who symbolize the world, who render into a shape that is conceptualized as the kind of material that can be worked over, then imagine that they can 'apply' their psychoanalytic knowledge to the world in such a way as to dispel the imaginary apprehension of social relations and burrow their way into the real. Not so, Lacanians. Lacanian psychoanalysts err, and know something of the way they must err in their understanding of the world, must knot together the symbolic, the imaginary, and the real in such a way that they cannot ever imagine that they have escaped the symbolic or claim that they really lay bare the real as infrastructure, the so-called base, as condition of ideology or as mere superstructure of contemporary society.

Oppression and resistance are threaded through every radical political theory and practice, and the contributions in this book provide different vantage points through which we can both symbolize the conditions of life that make psychoanalysis a viable option, a conceptual and practical resource for exploring and transforming subjectivity, and also situate our own psychoanalytic readings within the symbolic. Let's face it: psychoanalysis itself is enmeshed in the cultural phenomena it applies itself to, something that no amount of reflection on the entrails of 'countertransference' can enable us to escape. Psychoanalysis is but one symbolic system among others, a collection of competing 'lines of the symbolic' whose coordinates are given by the precise theoretical trajectory and training tradition of the analyst. The contributors to this book know that and assume responsibility for the positions they adopt in order to speak about the world.

The politics of psychoanalysis, which sometimes, it must be admitted, also takes the form of 'Lacanian ideology', demands that we position ourselves in relation to the forms of oppression that our clinical work so often unwittingly endorses and that we find ways to elaborate resistance that is productive, constructive; not reduced to what our poor analysands misunderstand about who they are or the forms of 'defence' they employ to keep themselves in their place. Resistance in this book is a properly political category, active engagement with the world in order to change it, and the contributors find different ways of turning psychoanalysis to the task of understanding the symbolic shape of oppression better to combat it.

Psychoanalytic clinical and theoretical work circulates through multiple intersecting antagonistic symbolic universes. This series opens connections between different cultural sites in which Lacanian work has developed in distinctive ways, in forms of work that question the idea that there could be single correct reading and application. The Lines of the Symbolic in Psychoanalysis series provides a reflexive reworking of psychoanalysis that transmits Lacanian writing from around the world, steering a course between the temptations of a metalanguage and imaginary reduction, between the claim to provide a god's–eye view of psychoanalysis and the idea that psychoanalysis must everywhere be the same. And the elaboration of psychoanalysis in the symbolic here grounds its theory and practice in the history and politics of the work in a variety of interventions that touch the real.

Ian Parker
Manchester Psychoanalytic Matrix

Introduction

Chris Vanderwees and Kristen Hennessy

> I see Lacan as a weapon of subversion against the current capitalist system: this capitalism of finance, dehumanized, with no people or subject, prone to slipping out of control. To be inspired by Lacan against this madness would be to sow disorder in order.
>
> (Badiou and Roudinesco 60–61)

How can Lacanian psychoanalysis help us rethink our theoretical, clinical, and cultural perspectives regarding intersections of politics, oppression, and resistance? As a psychiatrist and psychoanalyst, Jacques Lacan did not maintain any clear political leaning or invest in a publicly political stance. In conversation with preeminent historian of psychoanalysis Élisabeth Roudinesco, philosopher Alain Badiou acknowledges a "constitutive ambiguity" in Lacan's thinking whereby conservative ideas at times exist alongside an emancipatory radicality (Badiou and Roudinesco 26). Some psychoanalytic groups, for instance, have misconstrued and distorted Lacan's thinking on notions of symbolic law and the Name-of-the-Father, extending such distortions towards regressive and reactionary conservatism. Meanwhile, many progressive theoreticians, including Badiou, maintain that "Lacanian categories can be mobilized to understand, once more, an entire series of phenomena: The death throes of inherited hierarchies, the omnipresence of money, the constantly hurried and vain circulation of all things, and so on" (Badiou and Roudinesco 19). Such political ambiguity has led Roudinesco to characterize Lacan as an "apolitical" figure in her biographical depiction of him (115). Yet, to call Lacan apolitical is not especially nuanced given that he developed his thinking within a turbulent and revolutionary socio-political atmosphere while resisting what he understood to be the oppressiveness of the dominant psychoanalytic ideology of his era. Throughout his Seminars and other works, he engaged with the concerns of surrealists, communists, and anti-psychiatrists, as well as the developments of the sexual liberation movement, all while living through the Second World War and the revolutionary era of the 1960s in Paris. While he may not have sought a public

DOI: 10.4324/9781003212072-1

commitment to any particular party's cause, Lacan took a great interest in political matters and was active in his own project of resistance, which manifested as an opposition to the bureaucracy, authority, and standard frame of the International Psychoanalytic Association. He also challenged the field of ego psychology, critiqued the work of empiricist and positivist psychologists, and questioned the idea of a "whole self." Lacan's subject is a split subject. As a result, there is always a lack in the subject's desire and any notion of a "whole" always already has a hole in it. Further, any established conceptualization of "normal" becomes an *énorme mal* through its exclusions. Any institutional representation of "disorder" (psychological or otherwise) relies on a fiction of "natural order."

Lacan constantly challenged the psychoanalytic establishment, perhaps especially when he claimed controversially that no authority could actually authorize the psychoanalyst, but rather that the analyst must engage in a process of self-authorization. In this respect, Lacan undermined the authority of the psychoanalytic institution and its category of training analyst. He suggested that the analyst's endorsement of the analysand's identification with a part of the analyst or institution (introjection) could be considered misled and unethical insofar as such an approach may simply serve the imaginary assumptions, narcissism, and will to understand of the analyst but also could not possibly help the analysand to find their own desire. As such, Lacan advocated for an approach for working respectfully towards difference rather than sameness. He argued that the approach to analysis that aims to "strengthen the analysand's ego" could actually lead to the analyst's corroboration with the analysand's symptom. For Lacan, ego psychology too often encouraged the subject to conform or adapt to societal expectations of "normativity" and to identify with the analyst's "good" or "strong" parts of the ego. Lacan attempted to overthrow the idea of the clinician as an authority, an expert, or as the one who possesses a specialized form of knowledge about the patient and the patient's symptoms. For Lacan, the analyst knows nothing for certain and is only *supposed* to know so as to allow the transference to emerge while helping to facilitate the analysand's will to knowledge. In this regard, it is fundamentally the analysand who possesses knowledge of the symptom. Therefore, the analysand's discourse becomes the most important aspect of the direction of psychoanalytic treatment, which brings with it the expression and integration of subjective history, experience of truth in speaking over time, and eventual *savoir-faire* of the symptom through repetition compulsion in speech and the transference.

Psychoanalysis ought to help restore the analysand's voice. If there is a fundamental political act that occurs in Lacanian psychoanalysis, it is when the analyst helps to facilitate a radical space for the analysand to speak everything as freely as is possible. This sort of space for speaking can be liberatory and create space for difference on a subjective plane through free associations, lines of flight, and radical thought, all of which fundamentally resist a model or program that might encourage identification with the oppressor, that is, the clinician as authority. Lacan's approach to the clinic remains a radical conceptual reversal of the typical power relation between doctor and patient, where the doctor might interpret the symptom and the patient might identify or disidentify with the bestowal of such an authoritative interpretation. Of course, there can be no free association without some resistance, but Lacan emphasizes throughout his work that resistance is on the side of the analyst. It is the analyst's task to maintain such a radical conceptual reversal of the typical clinical power relation in allowing the patient to speak everything that comes to mind while not resisting but rather listening to the symbolic of what the patient has to say. The "talking cure" of psychoanalysis aims towards subjectification rather than objectification so that the analysand may discover their own voice and desire. What Lacan drew great attention to in clinical psychoanalysis is the power relations at work in the clinic within the dynamics of speech and rhetoric between the analyst and analysand. What he offered was a revolutionary approach to rethinking clinical psychoanalysis in a "return to Freud" that conceptualized the human as a split subject of the unconscious, a subject split by its inevitable immersion in the symbolic realm of language and discourse. This is the subject of a drive fraught with unconscious needs, demands, and desires, but yet also a subject who speaks with a voice addressed toward an other and an Other: a speaking being.

Lacanian psychoanalysis emphasizes the singularity and fragmentedness of each subject and facilitates a process of subjectification for the analysand rather than attempt to "psychoeducate," "normalize," "regulate," or "adapt" the subject's ego to the environment, which would be to objectify with a clinical gaze and generalize the analysand's condition of suffering. It is in this approach to the clinic that Lacan drew parallels between himself and Lenin during the rhetorical performativity of his Seminars while also drawing parallels between Freud and Marx (Badiou and Roudinesco 20). Perhaps if socialism attempts to rethink and reverse hegemonic structures and discourses in attempts to redistribute power or surplus value, restoring a voice to people and communities over states and institutions, Lacanian psychoanalysis aims to reverse the hierarchies of the clinic, restoring a radical space for the subject to discover and exercise a voice while speaking about anything that comes to mind.

Yet, Lacan remained skeptical of revolutionary ideals, their circulation, and their crystallization in the social imaginary. Beginning in May 1968 in France, the social scene erupted with the student occupation protests against capitalism, consumerism, traditional authority, institutional hegemony, and American imperialism. There were mass public demonstrations in the streets. More than 11 million workers of France's trade unions went on strike while protestors clashed with police. The cultural production of revolutionary sentiments and actions of the time led the French economy to a standstill over the course of several weeks. The intense period of unrest struck fear into political leaders, who began to worry about the possibility of civil war, outbursts of violence, and revolution. President Charles de Gaulle briefly fled France for Germany. Following a national election held in June, de Gaulle was later succeeded by Georges Pompidou, who continued to promote the Gaullist movement as a moderate conservative. In December of 1968 at the Centre Universitaire de Vincennes, an experimental school established to respond to the academic consequences of the protests that had occurred only several months earlier, Lacan spoke to hundreds of students and uttered a now famous statement of cynical reasoning: "the revolutionary aspiration has only a single possible outcome of ending up as the master's discourse. This is what experience has proved. What you aspire to as revolutionaries is a master. You will get one" (Seminar XVII, 207). Here, Lacan suggested that the major obstacle to revolutionary projects arrives in a repetitive impasse where it may only be a matter of time before a new hegemonic power takes shape and emerges with fresh dynamics of oppression and resistance within the socio-political realm. Lacan's statement echoes a Foucauldian sentiment whereby oppositional power is understood to have the capacity to grow as exclusionary and oppressive as what it opposes. What Lacan might have been highlighting in his sentiment to the students is the inevitability of power relations between people insofar as new masters take the place of the old ones. Lacan himself did not know how to handle this impasse except through attempting to reject his own position as a master and dissolve his own school. Peter Starr writes that despite Lacan's insistence on such an impasse as well as his own resistance to assert a clear political alignment in terms of social progressivism, "the political and theoretical history of post-May France testifies again and again to the ease with which the field mapped out by Lacanian theory could be recharted in explicitly political, even revolutionary, terms" (38). We must not forget the significance of Lacanian thinkers who played crucial roles in the anti-psychiatry movement, including Félix Guattari, Gilles Deleuze, and Maud Mannoni; in the women's liberation movement, including Antoinette Fouque, Luce Irigaray, and Michèle Montrelay; in the French Maoist movement, including Jacques-Alain and Judith Miller; and in upheavals of critical and textual theory, including Roland Barthes, Phillippe Sollers, and Julia Kristeva. If Lacan did not provide any explicit alignment with liberation movements, surely his work lends itself to interventions within discussions on individual and collective dynamics of class, politics, oppression, and resistance.

Several important attempts to bring Lacan's discourse into conversation with ideology and the political realm can be found elsewhere in the excellent works of Slavoj Žižek, Yannis Stavrakakis, Samo Tomšič, and Andreja Zevnik, but their respective works take up cultural, historical, or ideological matters more deeply and sometimes can seem distant from the roots of psychoanalysis as a clinical practice. This is why we have tried to include a significant amount of work in this collection written from the perspective of not only critical theorists and political thinkers but also experienced clinicians. Lacan engaged with ideas of various academic fields, including psychology, philosophy, linguistics, sociology, anthropology, sexuality studies, and mathematics, but did so as a psychoanalyst who maintained the importance of psychoanalysis as a discipline, one distinct from not only psychology and psychiatry but also philosophy. Lacan maintained a position not simply as a psychoanalyst but as an anti-philosopher, that is, critical of structural systems of thought that provide frameworks for institutionalized truths and dogmatic scientism, which can only inevitably lead to exclusion, censorship, oppression, and repression. Lacan's own discourse remains open and resists reduction to an easily explainable or digestible theory. Perhaps this is also why it holds great potential for rethinking our contemporary political state of affairs and continues to draw interest for a new generation. He importantly challenged the assemblages that sustain our impression of sociopolitical reality and have a bearing upon the subject of the unconscious. It is Lacan, through Freud, who provides us with a revolutionary approach to the human subject. The anti-philosopher also proposed an important dimension that exceeds any philosophy's horizon: the real. In Lacanian thinking, the real is traumatic, inexpressible, inaccessible, or unaccountable in any social, political, or individual discourse. It is the very subversive dimension of Lacan's real that each of the authors of the following chapters attempts to work through in contemporary cultural, theoretical, and clinical contexts.

In "Lacanian Psychoanalysis and Marxism: Conceptual and Practical Work," Ian Parker provides a manifesto for movements of liberation for a better world, which involves the interrelationship between the miserable exploitative oppressive reality of life today and our "internal" lives, our psychology. Psychoanalysis grasps that intimate interconnection between this reality and what feels deep within each of us. This chapter proposes that we must understand the nature of that interconnection to build a practical alternative to capitalism, sexism, and racism. Our task is to reconstruct psychoanalysis as an authentic form of "critical psychology" with the help of ideas gathered in the Marxist political–intellectual tradition and in the extensive theoretical and practical work carried out for a century at the intersection between Marxism and psychoanalysis. Parker addresses the role of the unconscious, repetition, drive, and transference in clinical and political analysis in order to address questions of subjective transformation.

In "Capital's *Jouissance*: Society and Sexual Political Economy in Lacan's Marx," David Pavón-Cuéllar explores how Lacan incorporates sexuality in his reading of Marx's critical approach to political economy. Pavón-Cuéllar examines how this reading allows Lacan to consider the role of enjoyment (*jouissance*) in exchange and use values, reconceptualizing them as enjoyment-value and enjoyment of value. He analyses how Lacan, resignifying psychoanalysis and not only Marxism, emphasizes the political character of

Freud's sexual economy. After examining how the relationship of the sexual with the social has been considered among various Freudian Marxist authors, he discusses some of Lacan's ideas about the sexual–economic foundation of society. He analyzes the way in which these ideas, preceded by Jean Audard and based on Claude Lévi-Strauss, connect Marxist and Freudian concepts by founding society on the patriarchal exploitation of women. Patriarchy, according to Lacan, reaches not only its apogee in capitalist modernity but also its crisis that manifests itself symptomatically through the discoveries of Marx and Freud. He attempts to explain why Marxism and psychoanalysis constituted for Lacan the last strongholds of the subject, of use value, and of knowledge in an increasingly automated capitalist system governed by exchange value and dominated by data and information. After glimpsing how capital monopolizes enjoyment in modern capitalist society, Pavón-Cuéllar notes that one must assume an enjoyment of capital to understand the Lacanian formulations in which exchange-value operates as enjoyment-value, use-value as enjoyment of value, and surplus-value as an expression of a surplus-of-enjoyment (*plus-de-jouir*), defined as the renunciation of enjoyment in the widespread discontent in culture. These formulations will help to outline the way in which Lacan theorizes both Freud's sexual economy and sexuality as a principle of the social.

In "Can We Decolonize Lacan?," Clint Burnham argues that we need a reading of psychoanalysis, qua its canonical texts but also a genealogy of its concepts, in terms of not only its colonial conditions (as Said takes up Freud) – for instance, what is the Algerian context for Lacan's discussion of Antigone? – but also in terms of the racialized or colonizing tropologies and significations that appear in Lacan (as Beshara argues with respect to Žižek). In what way does Lacan's "split subject," for instance, extract from Lévi-Strauss' misreading of Northwest Coast (Kwakiutl) transformer masks? Second, Burnham argues that we need to not shy away from drawing on psychoanalytic theory to think in a decolonial way. This chapter brings our attention to two contradictions of current decolonial theory and practice. First, the tension between decolonization and its relation to Indigenization (worked out in some ways by Tuck and Yang, Betasamosake Simpson, A. Simpson, and Glenn Coulthard) in ways that are coded as either identity politics (hiring demands in the academy, etc.) or authenticity discourses (land and sovereignty) in a way resistant to a decolonial cosmopolitanism. From here, Burnham opens up a new question: what does decolonial lack look like? If the goal is not some fantasy of authentic subjectivity, what is a decolonial split subject – beyond the obvious (but which should not be disavowed) splits and *métissage* and hybridity? Burnham considers, in particular, recognition, what we might even call a fear of recognition (in the guise of critique) on the Indigenous left (Coulthard) – not only working it back to Fanon (and Charles Taylor, as Coulthard does), Kojève/Hegel, and 1950s Lacan, but also thinking of how recognition becomes more structural in

Lacan, that moment in the mid- to late fifties (from the "Rome discourse" to the "Agency of the Letter," but also the Seminar on the formations of the unconscious) when his theorizing moves from the master/slave and other towards grappling with the big Other and the signifier. Burnham posits that theoretical progress – which in orthodox readings of Lacan then is "filled in," as it were, with the turn to formulas of sexuation and "there is no sexual relation" – can also be seen in terms of such colonial themes as the hysterical-decolonial subject, day schools/residential schools as unconscious/university discourse, the name of the father qua colonial interpellation, and so forth.

In "Dwelling on the Direction of the Treatment for the Homeless Subject," Chris Vanderwees explores the lack of psychoanalytic literature on poverty and the political implications of this lack while providing a reflection upon the praxis of institutional psychotherapy and therapeutic community. This chapter highlights the clinical importance of therapeutic labor and open-ended psychoanalytic treatment in a therapeutic community while also trying to express how a psychoanalyst cannot defensively withdraw one's desire to listen in the face of people who are homeless and impoverished (which would only reveal the resistance of the analyst); the psychoanalyst can, however, deploy an ethics given some variations to the more "classical" psychoanalytic frame so that space can be facilitated for the homeless subject to be able to speak about their own suffering.

In "Psychoanalysis is Spoken Here: Analytic Ethics and the Talking Cure in the Delivery of Community Mental Health Treatment," Christopher Meyer examines psychoanalysis as a practice whose conditions of possibility depend upon the capacity to construct an address for the "unspeakable." Given the demands placed upon beginning practitioners to adhere to evidenced-based approaches to the suffering and discontents of speaking beings, this chapter addresses the ethical stance called for (an analytic one) in order to hold a space for work with, from, and on the unconscious in the community mental health clinic with individuals identified as experiencing "severity" – in the fields of addiction, the psychoses, and the so-called borderline. Far from being unresponsive to or beyond the scope of analytic practice, this chapter argues that psychoanalysis holds a space for the subject of the unconscious as it appears and insists beyond the worried well. Psychoanalysis adheres to unconscious formations as a way of evoking a subject's "truth" regarding what would necessarily remain unsaid, repressed, and radically censored. The analytic act aims at the evocation and constitution of a new position in relationship to suffering that addresses the causes of trauma. Building upon his experience working with addiction, psychosis, and severity, Meyer proposes not only the importance of maintaining this position within community mental health clinics that are not ostensibly devoted to providing psychoanalytic treatment (e.g., how to adhere to the analytic act and its ethics within non-psychoanalytic clinics?), but also that Freud's dream of "free clinics" enjoins us to work toward the creation of Freudian-Lacanian clinics constructed from the logic and experience of those they work with rather than claiming to apply a ready-made treatment to the subject or consumer. It is important that the talking cure not only "haunt" clinics whose treatments at times inhibit speech but also give the ghosts of psychoanalysis a chance to be re-articulated in our community mental health clinics.

In "The Engimatic Body and the Constitution of Immigrants' Identity and Subjectivity," Debora Kirschbaum Nitkin explores how the experience of immigration may drastically disrupt and complexify one's experiences of the body. It exemplifies the intrinsic disjunction between being and body, which may be obscured in Cartesian approaches, such as the current medical discourse and its emphasis on the biological body. This happens because immigrating involves shifts in lifestyle, cultural references and values, language use, allocation in the labor market, and interpersonal relationships that significantly affect one's subjectivity and identity. Sometimes, these changes are experienced in the level of the body through the formation of body manifestations. For example, research shows that Canadian immigrants' physical and mental health tends to decline after the five first years after their arrival to Canada, a phenomenon called the "Healthy Immigrant Effect." Kirschbaum Nitkin observes resonances of this phenomenon in her clinical work with new or established immigrants, who often complain about body manifestations, such as panic attacks, headaches, leg pain, skin, and gastrointestinal issues, whose onset they associate with the post-immigration event. Strikingly, many of these cases were first diagnosed as "unexplained medical symptoms," after medical tests excluded the presence of anatomic or physiological alteration. This finding overwhelms those individuals, baffling them with a strong sense of disbelief and mystifying them with a worry at not understanding the medical results. Combined, these feelings propel the newcomer to seek psychotherapy in search for a response about the "reality" of those body manifestations.

In "A Conversation on Psychoanalytic Work with Children in the System," the editors discuss Kristen Hennessy's practice with children who live in foster or adoptive care. The conversation revolves around Hennessy's thoughts on the clinician's role as a listener, the mirror stage, the father function and the question of diagnostic structure, and the importance of play in enabling children to articulate and possibly transform the symptom in the family system.

In "The Controlled Act of Psychotherapy in Ontario: A Lacanian Impasse," Sheila L. Cavanagh analyzes the impasse between the Lacanian psychoanalytic act and the legal definition of the Controlled Act of Psychotherapy enforced by the College of Registered Psychotherapists of Ontario (CRPO), Canada. The legal act is inclusive of psychodynamic therapies and is, as Cavanagh will argue, at odds with what Lacan calls the psychoanalytic act. The Controlled Act of Psychotherapy includes a focus on 'diagnosis', 'impairment', 'outcomes', predetermined 'goals' and 'plans', along with clear distinctions between 'beginnings' and 'endings'. In Lacanian praxis, the psychoanalytic act involves desire (as opposed to diagnosis), a distinction between 'acting out' (for the Other in a given/repetitive scene) and a passage to the act (*passage à l'acte*) whereby the subject exits the Symbolic scene. The CRPO focus upon controlling the act is at odds with the psychoanalytic cure, the desire and discourse of the Lacanian analyst.

In "Groups and Communality: A Real Conundrum for the Social World," Eve Watson explores the organization of the psychoanalytic group, that is, the notion of a group that aims to support the work of analysts. A psychoanalytic group must support an insoluble paradox by incarnating the communal aims of analysts who are individually marked by the singularity of their relation to *jouissance* and the empty cause that is their lack-in-being. The drive cannot be shared or communally divided up. What is the social work that a psychoanalytic group must do to support the lack-in-being that defines each of its members, while facilitating the transmission of psychoanalysis? It is via a focus on the imperative to work and the assumption of the analyst's responsibility for their desire and surplus enjoyment. The neglect of each of these causes psychoanalytic groups to be exclusionary and elitist by producing a blind spot that ideology and politics comes to occupy. Watson suggests that the taint of elitism has dogged psychoanalysis since its inception, and this chapter assesses this in terms of the problematics of the psychoanalytic group itself.

In "A Spectral Materialism to Safeguard Modernity," Alireza Taheri takes up the question of ghosts, spirits, and specters, which typically belong to the domain of pre-modern superstition and are often thought to have no place in modern thought. According to Foucault, the classical period is inaugurated by Descartes' fateful decision to bar madness from discourse. In a different but related gesture of exclusion, Kant warned against reason's conceit to confront metaphysical questions (e.g., free will and determinism, the divisibility of matter). For Kant, the attempt to delve into these noumenal matters leads to the impasse of the antinomies of reason. Thought would henceforth have to limit itself to the sober domain of science defined as the study of phenomena, how things appear rather than how they are in-themselves. In this chapter, Taheri argues that these two measures of exclusion, intended to protect and guarantee the advent of the modern, paradoxically lead to the failure of modernity's full realization. The inaugural exclusion by which modernity attempts to establish itself leads to a return of the repressed compromising modernity's advance. Such resurgences of the pre-modern within our contemporary late modernity are attested to by the rise of New Age spirituality, the proliferation of new religiosities, the obscurantism of modern American psychiatry, and the mystical faith in the "invisible hand of the market." By contrast to the Cartesian marginalization of madness and the Kantian banishment of the noumenal, Hegel, Marx, and Freud dare to grant attention to these tabooed objects relegated to pre-modernity. Taheri argues that it is only by returning to these forsaken objects through Hegel (God), Marx (the mysticism of the commodity) and Freud (the dream) as well as other "spectral" entities (in Derridian parlance) that modernity can forge for itself an unshakable materialism immune to resurgences of pre-modern superstition.

In "Invisible Fist of the Market: *Fight Club* and the Therapeutic Lures of Violence," Daniel Adleman provides an exploration of Chuck Palahniuk's *Fight Club*, which he suggests is often misrecognized as an orgiastic celebration of hypermasculinist proto-incel violence, whereas the novel might actually best be understood as a much more nuanced, politically relevant interrogation of conventional understandings of violence. Far from blithely celebrating what Slavoj Žižek calls the "subjective violence" of fight clubs, the novel documents its nameless protagonist's therapeutic pilgrim's progress to sublimate the systemic violence of post-Fordist neoliberal capitalism and channel it in politically emancipatory directions. This chapter tracks the psychoanalytic dimensions of his increasingly entangled therapeutic and activist strategies to metabolize and wield what he explicitly characterizes as the castrating paternal violence of corporate-colonized America. His ever-unfolding odyssey to save himself and others (through his experiments with terminal disease self-help groups, fight clubs, anti-corporate activism, and ultimately terrorism) does far more than underscore the role of violence in late capitalist society; more importantly, Palahniuk's account of this therapeutic journey models a crucial set of optics on the relationship between a class-focused view of social justice and pivotal psychoanalytic concepts like resistance, acting out, passage to the act, psychosis, symbolic castration, the Law of the Father, and the big Other. The resulting framework begets political-psychoanalytic insights that Adleman brings to bear on both contemporary peaceful protest movements (including Occupy Wall Street and Idle No More) and the dispersed violence of social calamities (like "frictionless" digital capitalism, the incel movement, and the Covid-19 pandemic).

In the final chapter, "Self-Removed: Trauma, Irony and Animals," Bo Earle takes up the notion of trauma as a collapse of cultural meaning that entails a crucial but underappreciated loss of irony. To sustain a distinct cultural reality requires what thinkers from Lucretius to Hegel to Maus and Freud have variously characterized as "*symbolic excess*." That is, cultural meaning becomes a real world if the value we show it exceeds that of mere survival. As nomadic buffalo hunters, the Crow developed the practice of "counting coups" as a way of maintaining temporary yet indisputable proprietary claims to hunting territory. According to Jonathan's Lear account in *Radical Hope: Ethics in the Face of Cultural Devastation*, it is precisely the symbolic excess of this practice that creates Crow territory as an indisputable reality. It is remarkable that the term "counting coups" applies equally to the act itself of challenging enemies and subsequent ceremonial honoring of this act: as if accomplishing an heroic deed were on some level one and the same as being honored for such a deed, underscoring the importance of symbolic excess for the construction of cultural reality. The ultimate purpose of the deed is not just to ward off invaders but to perpetuate cultural meaning as an end in itself, to sustain a cultural reality. According to Lear, overcoming this collapse of Crow reality, or cultural devastation, requires inventing new ways of insisting on symbolic excess. Earle explores the Crow practice of "counting coups" as a remarkably non-proprietary, non-predatory, and non-consumerist model of cultural meaning and subjectivity. This is arguably a sense in which the Crow reality based on the chickadee as representative of a progress of sorts over the buffalo-based one; but the historical contexts of the two are so distinct that any evaluative comparison seems tendentious. Yet, as Lear mentions, given our own preoccupation with cultural devastation and various forms of apocalypse (by global warming, terrorism, etc.), the chickadee's wisdom seems potentially, particularly, instructive *to us now*. This chapter explores if and why such ironic wisdom must be mediated by an animal.

As a final word, let us highlight that Lacan demonstrated the political gesture in the form of disbandment, which can be observed in his associations and disassociations over time with various psychoanalytic groups in addition to the dissolution of his own school in 1980. What Badiou underscores about Lacan is the emphasis on an avoidance of the imaginary group effect. Badiou asks, "what does avoiding the group effect consist of? It consists of proposals of permutation, nonhierarchical stabilization, lability or changeability of everything, and putting an end to consistency as the duration of the group" (128–129). For Lacan, the ultimate political act is not "the foundational chartering of a collective nor the sovereign suspension of its laws, but the act of *dissolving* a group as such" (Reinhard xxxiv). Badiou's Lacan lays out the political path of the psychoanalyst as an imperative to disband:

> a political organization is always contingent and temporary; it has a task to accomplish rather than a status quo to prolong, and the authentic political decision is the determination of the proper moment to liquidate the political structure that has served its purpose.
>
> (xxxiv)

The authors of this collection have come together as a group to think through pressing contemporary political concerns inside and outside the clinic. If such a publication can be thought of as a foundational moment, let this moment also be a simultaneous dissolution as we disperse to take up these lines of flight elsewhere in the future.

Works Cited

Badiou, Alain. *Lacan: Anti-Philosophy 3. 2013*. Trans. Kenneth Reinhard and Susan Spitzer. New York: Columbia University Press, 2018.

Badiou, Alain, and Élisabeth Roudinesco. *Jacques Lacan, Past and Present: A Dialogue*. Trans. Jason E. Smith. New York: Columbia University Press, 2014.

Reinhard, Kenneth. "Introduction to the Seminar on Lacan." In Badiou, Alain. *Lacan: Anti-Philosophy 3*. Trans. Kenneth Reinhard and Susan Spitzer. New York: Columbia University Press, 2018. xxiii–xxxvii.

Roudinesco, Élisabeth. *Jacques Lacan*. 1993. Trans. Barbara Bray. New York: Columbia University Press, 1997.

Starr, Peter. *Logics of Failed Revolt: French Theory after May '68*. Stanford: Stanford University Press, 1995.

Chapter 1

Lacanian Psychoanalysis and Marxism

Conceptual and Practical Work

Ian Parker

Introduction

I am going to examine the connection between Lacanian psychoanalysis and Marxism through the lens of a joint book project with David Pavón-Cuéllar designed to make psychoanalytic arguments accessible to the left, that is, to articulate psychoanalysis with the practice of left movements. That book's title, *Psychoanalysis and Revolution: Critical Psychology for Liberation Movements*, expresses the broadest scope of the project; we are addressing activists in a number of different movements, ranging from explicitly anti-capitalist groups to ecological, indigenous and feminist networks, and we are using the signifier 'critical psychology' strategically to speak about psychoanalysis. We are concerned with practice, here political practice, but we know that there is no direct unmediated practice as such, that it must be mediated, explicitly or implicitly, by a theory of the world and a theory of the human subject. If it is not explicit, reflected upon and worked through, then that mediation is usually, by default, ideological.[1]

The conceptual underpinnings of the project are more specific than the title of the book indicates because of the theoretical and practical commitments we both have to Lacan and Marx. I frame this examination of the connection between the two as Lacanian psychoanalysis and Marxism, which is a little different from anchoring the work in the writings, pronouncements or, worse, supposed intentions of two authors. Lacan and Marx are, of course, at the core of this, and all the more so because the two traditions – of clinical practice and political practice – obsessively return to what is present, or absent, in these writers' texts.

There are innumerable contradictory readings of the possible relationship, and non-relation, between the two that cannot be settled by dividing the texts by way of 'epistemological breaks' or 'early, middle and later' stages of their work, or by even more precise minute divisions that will arrive at what version of each we should then articulate with what version of the other. We need, rather, to attend to how the anchoring of Lacanian psychoanalysis in Lacan and of Marxism in Marx operates, and this must be part of our work when we refer to what each are saying, ostensibly about the other.

DOI: 10.4324/9781003212072-2

Recuperation

This examination is primarily for Lacanians. It would look different if it were for Marxists. But there is an underlying problem that faces both of them, both of us, which is, again, to do with nature of the link between theory and practice. To make something 'accessible' – here in this project to make psychoanalysis accessible to the left – is always to risk banalising it. To some extent, that banalisation is inevitable.

With respect to Marxism, it means tackling the recuperation of the theory, the neutralisation and absorption of it by the very ideological forces it pits itself against, notably the ruling ideas that are the ideas of the ruling class.[2] The banalisation includes turning Marxism into a form of ideology, which is also exactly what it became as warrant for the bureaucracies in the temporarily 'post-capitalist' Stalinist workers' states. That ideologisation, then, has profoundly practical effects, giving rise to forms of 'Marxism' that are antithetical to what I would understand by it, antithetical to anti-Stalinist revolutionary Marxism.

I mark my position on this now so we can avoid some tendentious Lacanian readings of Marx later on. David will have a different political slant on this, but we Trotskyists and Maoists can bury our differences when need be, if not in the way that Stalin and Mao buried Trotskyists. The point is that misappropriation of Marx is materially effective; the ideological reformatting of Marxism becomes part of the conditions of possibility, and impossibility, Marxists encounter for political action. We could say that this ideologisation can be countered by critique and by 'praxis' – the dialectical interweaving of theory and practice – but that is easier said than done.[3]

This problem of banalisation makes things even more difficult for Lacanians. For psychoanalysis, as a theoretical framework that has been thoroughly recuperated by popular culture, banalisation is the name of the game, something we confront in our clinical practice when it takes form as a series of defences against the work. Lacan knew this. He had faced it as a material force incarnated in the International Psychoanalytical Association from which he had to break, and this is precisely why he is, as they say, so 'difficult' to read. That 'difficulty' does not solve the underlying problem, which is that we hold to this specific theoretical framework for psychoanalysis in the context of globalised processes of 'psychologisation' in which psychoanalytic culture plays a potent role, feeding specifications for subjectivity that are then lived out, experienced as interpersonal and intrapersonal reality. It is not surprising that these conditions of possibility and impossibility for psychoanalysis, an impossible profession, should work their way into the way practitioners as well as clients, analysts as well as analysands, understand and then attempt to theoretically elaborate what they are doing in the clinic, in their clinical practice.[4]

Metalanguage

We distrust commonsense operating in the line of the Imaginary, and the cultural conditions that give it a particular form, structured in the register of the Symbolic. And we Lacanians suspect that part of the problem is that commonsense invites us, tempts us, to imagine that we can rise above the ineliminable contradictions of the Symbolic so that we may then imagine that we are able to speak of such things as if within a metalanguage. Lacan famously declared that no metalanguage can be spoken, but this was after acknowledging, a few years earlier, that all language implies a metalanguage.[5] How can we square these two statements, that there is no metalanguage that can be spoken and that all language implies a metalanguage? There is a reflexive torsion in language that enables, even requires, it to speak of itself, but that does not mean that the many different sideways perspectives on the language we speak can be resolved into one god's-eye view of what exactly the language is as such, or what it is doing.

There is also a tension, which takes the form of an experiential paradox, between what can be spoken and what can be written, formalised in some way. It is an experiential paradox precisely because the truth that is spoken in psychoanalysis as a talking cure, truth of the subject that is both fleeting and liberating, can take shape as if it thereby operates as a metalanguage. On the side of the analysand, there is a particular temptation: the turning of what has been said by themselves in the transference or, worse, by their analyst, into a revelatory guide for life and an evangelical attachment to psychoanalysis. On the side of the analyst, there is a corresponding temptation; the idea that it is their interpretation that has made a difference and then they enjoy the sedimentation of that in reports of the case to colleagues. Then it is as if a metalanguage has been spoken.[6]

But if no metalanguage can be spoken, as Lacan claims, and I think he is correct here, is it also the case that no metalanguage can be written? This, I think, is a moot point, and it would seem, from both the privilege that Lacan accords writing as a domain of representation of psychoanalytic theory that is 'tighter' than speech and the activity of psychoanalysts' own writing, even before the attempted reduction of meaning effects in the 'mathematisation' of Lacanian psychoanalysis, that it can. That is perhaps why I needed to write this, even though it is possible for a written text to mimic speech and it is equally possible, and usually is the case for obsessional neurotic speech in analysis to be like writing, for there to be what Jacques-Alain Miller calls 'the written in speech'.[7] In some contexts, when the analyst suspects that there is psychotic clinical structure present in the clinic, one of the markers of which is the cursed ability of the analysand to witness the mechanics of the language they speak, there will be encouragement to write. Science itself, Jacques-Alain Miller, suggests in an early paper, is effectively psychotic.[8]

In other words, writing is the domain in which we find metalanguage, which is also one of the defining characteristics of most theoretical work, including about the psychoanalytic clinic. This is very different from speech in the clinic, which is where we will hear the truth of the subject, which is not, of course, empirical observable fact, not verifiable through the written analytical procedures of science. Perhaps that is why Lacan tries, according to Bruce Fink, to track a path somewhere between speech and writing, knowing well the importance of each domain of representation.[9] If writing is privileged in one domain, psychoanalytic theory, then speech is privileged in the other, the psychoanalytic clinic.

Writing that builds and sustains the architecture of our tradition of work does, of course, have a history. There are quite specific conditions of possibility for writing to appear on the world stage and quite specific subjective effects. Psychoanalytic writing 'mirrors', as it were, the emergence of what has been called 'print capitalism', a form of writing that configures what Benedict Anderson terms 'imagined communities' within nation states that developed in the couple of centuries following the fifteenth-century invention of the Gutenberg press.[10] A transformation of the Symbolic thus hosts the formation of specific forms of the Imaginary and specifications for and fantasies about what is Real. A range of other mediations of the Symbolic, including the 'Discourse Networks' account by Friedrich Kittler also has consequences for the way psychoanalysis has taken shape and been reshaped in the popular imagination.[11]

Here we begin to edge onto the domain of social-theoretical analysis of what makes psychoanalysis possible as a practice, and so onto the unnecessary but potent turf war between psychoanalysis and Marxism. Historical sensitivity to every form of practice, including its own, is one aspect of Marxism that attracted Lacan, and the battleground between Lacan and Marx has often revolved around the precise points where Lacan adapts Marxist theory and reformats it in line with his own attempt to analyse the cultural-historical conditions in which psychoanalysis functions; this most notably appears in the rewriting of Marx's category of 'surplus value' as 'surplus *jouissance*' and in his description of the 'four discourses' as structures that do indeed, Lacan insisted, march in the streets, that is, have a materially effective political existence.[12]

The problem is that these translations of concepts from the context of one frame into another then twists the relation between Lacanian psychoanalysis and Marxism from admiration and utility to rivalry and colonisation. Into the gap that opens up between the two then flood false oppositions that obscure both similarities and differences, and accusations that need to be carefully disentangled if we are to go any way towards closing the gap again. Marxist Lacanian psychoanalysis could then really still be Lacanian. Let us turn, first, to the similarities between the two traditions to be clear about the grounds of the debate between them.

Similarities

We need to separate out different aspects of similarity between Lacanian psychoanalysis and Marxism and to attend to the way each apparent similarity includes a twist, something that doesn't quite correspond to what the putative rival partner is up to. Here are five.

Suspicion

First is the well-known indexing of Freud and Marx, and Nietzsche, as 'masters of suspicion', a characterisation of a particular approach to hermeneutics provided by Paul Ricoeur.[13] This is a characterisation that has taken in social theory, both as a way of grasping these figures as critical inheritors of the Western Enlightenment, beyond a hermeneutics of faith, and as setting them up as masters to be deposed by later supposedly non-interpretative immanentist theorists. The twist here is that both Marx and Lacan actually go further in their versions of the 'hermeneutics of suspicion' than they are usually given credit for in the popular imagination and in mainstream psychoanalytic debate.

In Marx's case, this sets him against conspiratorial accounts of the social, even though Marxism is often confused with such toxic political approaches. Capitalism is not bad because of bad people making money and pulling the strings to protect their property. Marxism pits itself against systemic corruption in which 'surplus value' is a marker of the problematic nature of social relationships. The question is not how to redistribute 'surplus value' more fairly, but how to overthrow a political-economic system structured by the accumulation and investment of surplus value in the form of the 'universal equivalent', money as a commodity.

In Lacan's case, a hermeneutics of suspicion sets him against depth psychology, even though psychoanalysis is often reduced to that. The ego is not bad because it is mistaken about what lies beneath it, learning about hidden motives so it may become more flexible and adaptable. Lacanian psychoanalysis pits itself against attempts to tame *jouissance*, but not thereby in order to release it, as would be the aim of many Freudo-Marxists.[14] The question is not how to lift repression but rather to track how the repression operates. The question concerning 'surplus *jouissance*' is not how to spend it sensibly but, as *objet petit a*, to map its effects.

So, in both cases, a hermeneutics of suspicion leads these two theorists to also be suspicious about the function of reductive attempts to discover what is secretly guiding or driving their object of study, whether that is capitalism that Marxism aims to overthrow, or the 'subject of science' that Lacanian psychoanalysis works upon, of which more below. In both cases, those reductive explanations that they avoid are precisely part of the problem, false explanations that must be addressed in the course of analysis.

They complement each other when working in their own domain, and they clash when they stray from it. The suspicion of conspiracy-theoretic explanation and depth psychology warns the Marxist off trying to account for why certain political figures behave as they do and warns the Lacanian off trying to 'analyse' these political figures. At least, it should warn them off, for the warning is not always heeded.

That is when they clash, one instance of which is when surplus *jouissance* is vaunted by Lacanians as being an 'equivalent' of surplus value, when there is a slippage from treating each form of surplus as serving a function in the political economy of capitalism or the psychic economy of the bourgeois subject. That is also when we begin the fruitless task of explaining to Marxists what surplus value really is, as 'Marxlust', Marx's own surplus enjoyment, for example.[15] Needless to say, neither can the enigmatic non-empirical nature of the *objet petit a* be explained in Marxist terms as a simple accumulation of 'profit' for the subject. Each reductive interpretation of what the other means is misplaced.

Change

The second similarity revolves around the intimate necessary link between analysis and transformation. A hermeneutics of suspicion makes both of the traditions of work perfectly suited to an academic enterprise, at home in the university, dispensing interpretations as currency of the institution and accumulating knowledge. The actual nature of analysis, in both cases, political analysis or personal analysis, however, is antithetical to the university. This, on two counts; interpretations are 'mutative', they are designed to change what they analyse, and interpretations are produced by the subject themselves, not by an accredited knowledge-monger.[16] But here is a twist, which concerns the nature of the 'subject' of change.

For Marxism, the subject is formed in the interpretative revolutionary process as a collective subject, but even then 'divided', we might say. The analysis that is impelling and informed by the change that is happening is contested, as contest between different social actors and as contradiction running through them. This contestation is conceptualised by Marxists as being 'dialectical', internally coherent but contradictory, mutating, even turning into its opposite. And the division in the collective subject is conceptualised, after the event, in terms of which class elements play a vanguard role and which function as avatars of reactionary class interests. The vanguard is not the Leninist Party inserting correct analysis from the outside but is rather the collective subject of revolutionary change reconfiguring itself as proletariat, demanding change in the conditions it now identifies as hindering it; its own analysis of its predicament entails the revolutionary overthrow of capitalism.[17]

For Lacanian psychoanalysis, the speaking subject in the clinic appears as if it is unitary, undivided, but its truth, Lacan reminds us, is always 'half-said'.[18] It is, at one moment, 'individual' in the sense of being separate, standing alone, singular, working through the clinical process as something that proceeds 'one by one'. But it actually disrupts the sense of 'individual' as being something undivided; what it speaks may or may not correspond with what it hears itself say. Interpretation that strikes a chord in the subject and opens it up to change, to a transformation in its relation to the Symbolic, is not something that can come from the analyst; it must come from the analysand. It is as the analysand analyses that they transform who they are.

In neither case, then, is interpretation offered from outside the subject, and certainly not in the form of ready-made knowledge that has been accumulated and tried and tested. Each transformative moment, whether it is in the clinic or on the political stage, is singular, and each operates through a break with the fantasy of a metalanguage, whether that is a metalanguage about normative development or about stages of history. What knowledge there is about change is not within the accepted frame of neutral 'academic' language, but rather a guide to action, and then usually elaborated after the event.

Here is another reason why it is not permissible for one field of action to operate as a metalanguage in relation to the other. Here again is another warning against offering, from within one domain, an interpretation that pretends to clarify what is being elaborated in another. The domain of the collective subject, the subject of politics for Marxism, is qualitatively different from the domain of the individual subject who speaks in analysis. The transformative moments when these very different divided agential phenomena appear as subjects are not only specific to the domain in which they operate as a theoretical-reflexive break from the past, but they also cannot be completely confined within any one analytic frame. Something they share, which makes them all the more irreducible to analysis from outside, is that there is something excessive and unpredictable about the change they invite, require and provoke.

Knowledge

The third similarity concerns the nature of knowledge and well-founded reluctance to turn a theoretical frame, whether it is informing a clinical or political tradition, into a 'worldview'. We know that Lacan follows Freud's warnings about turning psychoanalysis into a worldview and Freud's insistence that the closest psychoanalysis comes to being a worldview is to the worldview of science.[19] This is not to say that psychoanalysis is part of the worldview of science; rather, it is the worldview psychoanalysis comes closest to. Lacan's precision of this argument is in the claim that psychoanalysis works on the subject of science.[20] That is a question that takes us to the historical specificity of the kind of subject psychoanalysis is geared to, to which we will return in a moment. Marxism has trod an unhappier path down this route, from the debates about whether there is a dialectics of nature to the formation of the bureaucracies in the temporarily post-capitalist states for which Marxism was, indeed, treated as a worldview; resistance to the bureaucratisation of Marxism has also entailed a critical reflection on the supposed nature of Marxism as a worldview.[21] It is not.

The task of analysis in each case is not to embed the subject in a worldview but to break them from it. But here is a twist, for alongside resistance to the turning of the theoretical frame itself into a worldview, there is a different evaluation of the nature of worldview as such and, more importantly, to the nature of the break.

For Marxism, such a break is imperative, built into the theory; it is a theory that is designed to speak for the working class, against capitalism from the standpoint of those who work, those who produce 'surplus value'. Or, better, and this is where we stay true to the transformative aspect of analysis, it speaks from the standpoint of an as-yet-to-be constituted proletariat as a universal subject.[22] It cannot be underestimated how crucial this wider dimension of the revolutionary process is, something expressed in suspicion of the possibility of constructing socialism in one country and insistence, instead, on the international dimension of political struggle.[23]

For Lacanian psychoanalysis, on the other hand, we do not, however much we set ourselves against the goal of adapting people to society, aim to break our analysands from anything. We hold no normative position about what kind of relationships will make them happy, or even moral evaluation of what happiness is or whether it is necessarily a good thing. The personal transformative change that occurs in the clinic one by one may or may not be visible to the analyst; in contradistinction to Marxism – for which the public collective nature of struggle is to be as visible as possible, to enrol the maximum number of subjects to it – Lacanian psychoanalysis enables some of the tiniest, most imperceptible changes and, indeed, is rightly suspicious of those who evangelise about it.

However much we dislike capitalism – and there is much useful Lacanian analysis critical of the discourse of the university and the contemporary malaise of civilisation that provides valuable insight into the personal misery concurrent with globalised consumerism – we Lacanians do not aim in our clinical work to overthrow it. The injunction to 'escape' capitalism, which is quite impossible while it still exists as a political-economic system, is, while being an individualist mimesis of Marxist politics, not strictly-speaking Lacanian at all.[24] Marx famously refused to sketch out a blueprint for what a post-capitalist society would look like, and that sensitivity to the problem of a worldview chimes with a Lacanian suspicion that the new world we may attempt to build for ourselves would simply replicate the world we think we have escaped. But Marxism does wager that another world is possible, one without surplus value, something that Lacanians would never dream of doing with respect to surplus *jouissance*.

History

The fourth similarity concerns the nature of history and the place of a theoretical framework designed to grasp it: the nature of history and its own place in that history. Simply put, both theoretical frameworks are reflexively attentive to the way they have developed at a certain point in history to address and work upon and transform a certain kind of subject. Actually, the link is closer than that because the two traditions of work emerged coterminously. This is one of the reasons they continually touch each other, impact on the work of the other, even treating the other as part of the problem. Each has had to disentangle itself from the sense that the other operates as a kind of mirror, in miniature or as projection, of the other, something neither has completely succeeded in doing.

Marxism emerges first not as a theory, as such, but rather as a critique of existing theories of political economy – Marx's *Capital* carries the subtitle 'a critique of political economy', not of capitalism, though it is that too – and it addresses a problem, capitalism, that is to be solved.[25] Then, just as Marxism came into existence with the birth of capitalism, working alongside the proletariat as the grave-digger of capitalism, the very grave-digger this political-economic system could not but create and nurture, so it will disappear when capitalism is finished. In other words, Marxism, despite the temptation to turn itself into a worldview in the hands of Stalinists, makes rare claim to provide a universal trans-historical theory, and when it makes such claims, it is quite un-Marxist.

Lacanian psychoanalysis, as we have already seen, reflexively positions itself as a historically emergent practice.[26] It too develops as a form of critique in two moments, first against psychiatry and then, as an internal critique, against the ego-psychological institutional apparatus of the International Psychoanalytical Association. And from that theoretical struggle comes an encounter with the nature of 'science' that the IPA was keen to find shelter with, and Lacan's analysis of the analysand as subject of science. The twist in this case concerns how we relate to the historical nature of the subject and the world that conditions its existence.

Marxism will not let go until it has destroyed capitalism, and it faces a world that should already have disappeared, but the contours of this world are – unfortunately for Marxist activists, though fortunately for Marxist theorists – if anything a replication of the political-economic conditions Marx analysed. They are even, with the even more intense globalisation of capitalism and its re-emergence on the territory of the old Stalinist states, operating as an exaggerated form of the world Marx described.

There are technological transformations such that we are well beyond the mutations analysed by Marxists of service-sector–heavy 'late capitalism' and the saturation of relations of production by consumerism, the economic pole of capitalism Marx did not himself have time to deal with.[27] However, the role, if not the precise nature of 'surplus value', is still very much in place, as is the ideological mystification of it. That ideological mystification is, if anything, more intense with the intensification of consumerism and the proliferation of simulacra of the cultural field. It provokes ideological fantasies of what is real and what is the core of human creativity, fantasies that circle around 'use value' as if that were the bare source and index of universal and essential human needs rather than the product of 'exchange value', historically located and mutable. Collective change is thus blocked at the very moment that the enigma of the intimate relationship between productivity and what is lost bewitches each individual subject.

Lacanian psychoanalysis, meanwhile, is beset by debate over the disappearance of the kind of subject that it aimed to treat, agonising over its place as a site of treatment for 'new symptoms', adapting itself to this intensification of consumerism and haunted by what remains of the human subject when so much of it is lost.[28] It is this that Lacan noticed and attempted to grasp when he invented the *objet petit a*, an object that operates as the site of surplus *jouissance*, that is at one moment alluring, excessively pleasurable, and at the very same moment impossible, haunting the subject as something lost.

It is exactly this 'surplus *jouissance*' that we find in the fantasies of 'use value' that drives subjects to find something beyond and beneath the shallow surface of commodity exchange. Lacan put his finger on something valuable for Marxist analyses of the nature of commodities but misidentified this surplus *jouissance* as equivalent, homologous to surplus value. We need to reorient Lacanian social theory to the nature of use value in order to better explicate how surplus *jouissance* as ideological place-marker of use value functions in the psychic and political economy of capitalist society.

Institutions

The fifth similarity concerns the institutional context for the two traditions and has some bearing on that last question, how one adapts one's practice to new conditions and how one lets go of analytic presuppositions that are out of date. This institutional question parallels the seepage of Marxist and psychoanalytic notions into contemporary commonsense, more in some cultural contexts than others, but throwing up obstacles as well as providing opportunities for adherents to gain followers. The consequence in both cases is, on the one hand, a degree of theoretical rigidity, which makes contact with the other tradition difficult, at best confused, and, on the other hand, proliferation of different readings of the founding texts such that we cannot always be sure which Marx and which Lacan we are talking about.

When we speak of Lacanian psychoanalysis and Marxism we are not, in fact, talking about fealty to the raw texts of each single author, an author who functions as the anchor of each tradition as master signifier, but allegiance to a reading of those texts refracted through particular institutions, most often institutions of the 'party' and the 'school'. And here is a paradox, and a twist in the relationship between the two traditions, which is that as each tradition that is so suspicious of recuperation, by academic institutions or the discourse of the university, struggles for survival, it has often either taken shelter in the university or mimicked the university in its own separate institution. This gives rise to a double problem, which is that the so-called debate between two such similar traditions of work is also refracted through the institutions that house it rather than the practice itself. It is this similarity, and only this one, that we can say is a homology. The other similarities, concerning interpretation, change, knowledge and history, operate as mere analogies.[29]

Marxism takes form in its revolutionary practice, a form that also often sabotages its practice, as a party. This is historically in the communist parties and, a necessary step, the formation of a communist international, which degenerated into a bureaucratic machine of state power in the Soviet Union in the early 1920s or into cognate organisations around the world that were turned into diplomatic instruments of Moscow. Attempts to resist this process by Marxists have often ended up repeating it in miniature, in ever-more rivalrous sectarian form. The party thus tends to replicate, in its notions of leadership and vanguard, exactly the forms of power and attachment to power that structure capitalist society, and it usually obsessively circles around the question of how to harness class forces that are operating independently of it, repeatedly implementing the same organisational procedures in quite different cultural and historical contexts, unable to master material and symbolic processes that escape its control.

Lacanian psychoanalysis typically institutes itself as a 'school' that attempts to escape the fate of the bureaucratised International Psychoanalytical Association, but that even so accumulates a cadre charged with governing training and transmission. Each attempt to break from this replication of the institution, of status, of the desire of the analyst, has failed.[30] We have seen, instead, a proliferation of different 'schools' and different international associations. This is despite psychoanalysis having close to hand the theoretical tools to critically reflect on this process, which are: a conception of transference that it extrapolates from the clinic but which it tends to exacerbate rather than dissolve; theories of the relation between desire and drive as being configured around that which operates through a claim for recognition and that which is quite meaningless activity; an understanding of the nature of this replication of forms through repetition; and, of course, of the nature of the unconscious, of what escapes every attempt of the institution to predict and control it.

This is the field on which we Lacanians usually pitch our battles, institutional battles for prestige that we call 'debate', including debate with rival theorists such as Marx. Not always; there are spaces that are more open, but they are hedged in by larger, more powerful institutional forces. It is then not enough, and is actually rather a distraction, to pretend that the similarities are what makes the debate worthwhile. We also need to attend to the supposed differences between the two traditions.

Differences

We can briefly identify four differences between Lacanian psychoanalysis and Marxism, some of which have been touched on already insofar as they emerge dialectically as twists in the apparent similarities between the two traditions. The questions, from a Lacanian point of view, might be whether these differences are 'Real', in the sense of functioning as an irreducibly antagonistic difference underlying and sabotaging anything that could be said of it by either side, Imaginary as aspects of rivalrous miscommunication or Symbolic as mediated by difference of theoretical frame.[31]

The question from a Marxist point of view is slightly different and here tends to circumvent that first 'real' obstacle that some Lacanians would identify when debating with Marxists; for some Marxists, those schooled in the Stalinist tradition in which their theory has become crystallised as a worldview, there might indeed be irresolvable doctrinal differences between them and Lacanians, and so the problem is a manifestation of a wish for doctrinal purity. It is here that the fifth ostensible 'similarity' between the two traditions, over the role of institutions that represent and transmit theory, is actually so problematic. For many Marxists, however, the question revolves around the reactionary or progressive function of rival theories they encounter, here whether Lacanian psychoanalysis assists, or complements, or obstructs class struggle, the struggle of the working class for power against material and ideological defence of capitalist property relations. We need to bear these issues in mind when we consider the differences, for they concern what really counts as a difference for each side.

Discontents

The first oft-cited difference revolves around the status of sexual repression as underlying what Freud described as the unease inherent in culture – what is usually glossed as 'Civilization and Its Discontents', following the English-language title of his book – and whether it is this or class struggle that should be viewed as primary.[32] Against the so-called Freudo-Marxist double-reduction – to natural sexual expression as the core driver of liberation and to the nuclear family in capitalist society as repressive enemy – Lacan argues that what we think of as 'sex' is operative in a number of fantasy-scenarios.

There is no possible sexual liberation, and so the task is to show how sexual difference, that which Lacan reconfigures as 'sexuation', is structured in class society. This, against those who would treat sexuation as the underlying bedrock of class struggle, who would then continue privileging psychoanalytic accounts, turning them into a reductive continuation of Freudo-Marxist theories. The question, then, is how 'sexuation' is either universalised or historicised.[33]

Conditions

The ideological reading of 'sexuation', reading it in line with bourgeois familial precepts about fixed sexual difference, versus a historical reading that asks how what is constructed can be deconstructed in progressive political practice, connects directly with the second key question dividing Lacanian psychoanalysis from Marxism: are we discussing and working with the human condition anchored in sex as unchangeable or tracking and facilitating mutations in the interpretation of biology by the human subject?

Alongside competing views about what is primary and secondary in human nature – what is the supposed bedrock and what emerges as our 'second nature' – are different standpoints on whether this or that obstacle to human liberation can ever be transcended.[34] Lacan's return to Freud resolves this question in favour of historical conditions of possibility and impossibility – it is that which underpins our ethical commitment to the possibility of change in our clinical practice – and this actually connects with Marxist accounts of the necessity for some notion of 'human nature' in our political practice.[35]

Collectivity

It would seem that the third difference, concerning whether analysis must proceed one by one, from the standpoint of the individual subject, or as a collective process through the constitution of a trans-individual subject, must pit Lacanians against Marxists. In practice, the question is whether such differences of domain – the domain of application of each form of analysis – need necessarily forbid the other. They need not.

From the Lacanian side, there is a multiplicity of accounts of the nature of the 'subject' that make it clear that this divided crux of human action is not necessarily mapped onto the individual body. Our Lacanian understanding of subjectivity is of it as being 'extimate', looping what is apparently exterior 'context' around what is ostensibly interior, and so when we speak of 'subject' we may do so in such a way as to include what is conventionally sociologically described as 'collective' as much as it is 'individual'.[36] This connects with rather than divides us from recent socialist-feminist readings of Marxism as including a political struggle over the nature of the separation between the 'personal' and the 'political'.[37]

Speech

The status of psychoanalysis as a 'talking cure' would seem, at first glance, to align it with what some Marxists would see as the superstructure rather than the material base of society, and so open up another chasm, another difference, between ideological if not idealist concerns, on the one hand, and materialist analysis and practice, on the other. This fourth difference is, however, as tendentious as the first three. The base–superstructure metaphor was, after all, a fleeting one within the Marxist tradition, inviting a series of crude reductive understandings of what is directly 'economic' and what is not. Again, it is the institutionalisation of Marxism in forms of Stalinism that is the problem, something that then unfortunately corresponds with the reduction of psychoanalysis to psychology among those in the IPA. The realm of the economic is not bedrock of political practice any more than a core self housed in the ego is in clinical practice.

Lacan's meditations on the nature of human action, and then 'act' in the clinic, have opened up new ways of thinking about what it means to speak well and how that is interwoven with covert or overt transformations of the Symbolic realm, a realm that is itself a material structuring force in political economy. There is no human subject without a symbolic structuring mediation between individuals, and Marxism is precisely concerned with how that mediation is politically–economically organised. In that sense, it is effectively Lacanian.

In each of these four cases, then, it would seem that despite the deep problem of political-ideological purity in the Marxist tradition, an institutional matter, it is actually the supposed purity and then intransigence of some evangelists for Lacanian psychoanalysis that is the problem, that creates obstacles to a fruitful encounter between the two sides. However, it is actually the Lacanian tradition that returns to Freud in such a way as to enable him to connect dialectically with Marx. We thus need to push at those conceptual edges of Lacanian theory grounded in its clinical practice.

Accusations and responses

It is in that light, in light of the failure to work through the differences, that we can address accusations made against Lacanians by Marxists and begin to assess whether those accusations are fair or misplaced, real concerns or expressions of misunderstanding or ideological confusion. It is certainly true that some Marxist complaints about psychoanalysis in general rest on specious arguments and false oppositions, oppositions that are treated as empirical universal givens rather than as dialectically structured; among such false oppositions, we can note that between what is material and what is ideal, between the so-called base and superstructure, and then between reality and mere language.

This way of proceeding leads to the most reductive and useless of oppositions, between what is proletarian and what is bourgeois, and then obscures the way that Lacanian psychoanalysis actually offers some way of working through those other oppositions.[38] A paradox is that Marxism can resolve those other oppositions in its own practice but usually fails to do so as an academic enterprise. Lacanian psychoanalysis cuts across those oppositions in its clinical practice but is restricted to that particular domain. It is not a theory or practice of politics. But this already anticipates accusations that are levelled against it by Marxists.

Such accusations include summarising and condensing into a list issues that have already been addressed so far: that psychoanalysis reduces politics to the level of the psychological; that change is reduced and confined to the level of the individual; that the clinical practice distracts from political practice, even presenting itself as an alternative to it; that the tragic central-European sensibility of psychoanalysis leads to irremediable pessimism about social change; that it absorbs insights about its shortcomings in such a way as to crystallise further its nature as a hermetic worldview in order to pathologise naysayers; that it professionalises care in such a way as to make it part of the apparatus of segregation and individualisation of distress; and that its institutions reinforce hostility to social forces that threaten to undermine their own privileged role as licensing interpretations of social ills.[39]

One sub-text of our book project on psychoanalysis, configured strategically as critical psychology for liberation movements is indeed a response to these accusations by Lacanians who are also Marxists. We do this by taking four fundamental psychoanalytic concepts – the unconscious as what is irremediably other to ourselves; repetition as the machine-like and contextually variable re-enactments of the past; drive as unbidden force and motor of self-sabotage and transformation; and transference as but one name for power relations in the clinic – and showing how each is actually grounded in political struggle.

Although we do not claim or believe that every authentic liberation movement, whether that is anti-racist, indigenous, post-colonial or feminist must be Marxist, the way we articulate our understanding of political struggle is, of course, underpinned by Marxism. And so, there is a double underlying argument running through the book, which is that Lacan is an invaluable conceptual resource for radicals who are willing to embrace psychoanalysis, and that Marx is an invaluable political compass point for psychoanalysts linking up with liberation movements. We think we can do this without declaring allegiance to particular institutionalised readings of Lacan in one particular school, and without deciding for one specific organisational current in Marxist theory and practice.

Conclusions

In some important respects, Lacan is wrong about Marx, with declaration as if by fiat and lured by a good pun, he mistakenly locates surplus *jouissance* as one of the forms of *objet petit a* in Marx's description of surplus value, rather than in the more alluring and insubstantial 'use value'. This then misleads a tradition of Lacanian psychoanalysis keen to trace out a supposed homology between Lacan's quite strategic description of the four discourses and Marx's critique of political economy. It is not that there is no homology between Lacanian psychoanalysis and Marxism; it is rather that, once it is itself absorbed into the academic-scholarly apparatus of the discourse of the university, Lacanian psychoanalysis looks for that homology in the wrong place, in the domain of theory as such rather than in the materialisation of that theory in the organisations that speak for it. In this way, the practice is refracted through institutional forms and through an apparently closed conceptual apparatus.

The apparent similarities between the two traditions of work thus obscure the specific contribution of each to our work, something that has dire sectarian consequences for any project that attempts to link psychoanalysis with revolutionary politics. We need to attend to the differences between the two traditions in such a way as to avoid false conceptual oppositions, and then be in a better position to respond to accusations made against us Lacanians by Marxists. We need to find a different way of speaking about the practice of each in relation to the practice of the other.

Marxism does in some sense need to also be Lacanian, but in such a way as to avoid the colonising impulse of a psychoanalytic tradition that too often reconfigures itself as a worldview. Lacanian psychoanalysis provides Marxism with an account of the unconscious, repetition, drive and transference in such a way as to avoid reductive and colonising depth-psychological accounts of the force and relations that enable and impede political action. That is why it underpins our conceptual and practice work on psychoanalysis as a form of critical psychology for liberation movements, a form of critical psychology that is not, as it turns out, not psychological at all. Here there are fruitful and necessary intersections between Marxism as a theory and practice of class struggle and anti-colonial, indigenous, anti-racist and feminist politics; here is a way of taking seriously the socialist-feminist slogan that the 'personal is political' without reducing one to another. There, in our book project, we effectively argue for a Lacanian conception of the subject – the human subject and agent of change – as a revolutionary force.

Lacanian psychoanalysis in our view is also in some important respects Marxist, but no less Lacanian for that. Lacanian psychoanalysis is a historically conditioned form of clinical practice that embeds the human subject in an account of language as that which exceeds it, treating the body, our material existence as human beings, as site of power, enigma and fantasy, a source of creativity that is both productive and lost. This is particularly so when this subject as subject of science is subject to surplus alienation as a function of the gap between use value and exchange value. Freud invented the unconscious, repetition, drive and transference as corollaries of the peculiar and inescapable alienation that structures our relation and non-relation with civilisation, and Lacan reconfigured these inventions in such a way as to render them as historical-materialist factors in clinical work. Though contained in the clinic, as a function of the clinic, these factors speak of the conditions of possibility that enclose them, and they operate dialectically in such a way as to link what we construct inside the clinic, the Lacanian task, with what we make of ourselves in the world, which is where we must speak of Marxism.

Notes

1 On critical psychology that intersects with psychoanalysis, see Parker, I. and Pavón-Cuéllar, D. (eds.) (2017) *Marxismo, psicología y psicoanálisis*. Morelia, Mexico: Paradiso editors, Universidad Michoacana de San Nicolás de Hidalgo.

2 For a nuanced account of this symbolic mediation that stresses the role of 'recuperation', see Debord, G. (1967/1977) *Society of the Spectacle*. Detroit: Black and Red.

3 On the praxis of contemporary Marxist theory, see Balibar, E. (2017) *The Philosophy of Marx*. London: Verso; Bensaïd, D. (2002) *Marx for Our Times: Adventures and Misadventures of a Critique*. London: Verso.

4 On psychologisation, see De Vos, J. (2012) *Psychologisation in Times of Globalisation*. London: Routledge; De Vos, J. (2013) *Psychologization and the Subject of Late Modernity*. London: Palgrave.

5 For 'all language implies a metalanguage', see Lacan, J. (1993) *The Seminar. Book III. The Psychoses, 1955–56*. Trans. Russell Grigg. London: Routledge, p. 226, and for 'there is no metalanguage that can be spoken', see Lacan, J. (1960) 'The Subversion of the Subject and the Dialectic of Desire in the Freudian Unconscious', in Bruce Fink (trans.) (2006) *Écrits*. New York: Norton, p. 688.

6 On the problematic transmission of 'truth' in the clinic, see Parker, I. (2018) 'Psychoanalytic Clinical Case Presentations, The Case Against', *Lacunae: APPI International Journal for Lacanian Psychoanalysis*, 17, pp. 6–36.

7 On writing and speech, see Miller, J-A. (1993) 'The Written in Speech', www.ch-freudien-be.org/Papers/Txt/Miller.pdf.

8 On science, see Miller, J-A. (1968) 'Action of the Structure', in P. Hallward and K. Peden (eds.) (2012) *Concept and Form Volume 1, Selections from Cahiers pour l'Analyse*. London: Verso.

9 On the tension between speech and writing in Lacan's work, see Fink, B. (2004) *Lacan to the Letter: Reading Écrits Closely*. Minneapolis: University of Minnesota Press.

10 On print capitalism, see Anderson, B. (1991) *Imagined Communities: Reflections on the Origin and Spread of Nationalism, Revised Edition*. London: Verso.

11 On discourse networks, see Kittler, F (1985/1990) *Discourse Network 1800/ Discourse Network 1900*. Stanford, CA: Stanford University Press.

12 On the four discourses, see Lacan, J. (1991/2007) *The Other Side of Psychoanalysis: The Seminar of Jacques Lacan, Book XVII* (translated with notes by R. Grigg). New York: W.W. Norton and Co.

13 On the 'masters of suspicion', see Ricoeur, P. (1965/1970) *Freud and Philosophy: An Essay on Interpretation*. New Haven: Yale University Press.

14 For an extended account of the different threads of this tradition and its shortcomings, see Pavón Cuéllar, D. (2017) *Marxism and Psychoanalysis: In or Against Psychology?* London and New York: Routledge.

15 For two accounts that take this line, see Bruno, P. (2020) *Lacan and Marx: The Invention of the Symptom*. London and New York: Routledge; Tomšič, S. (2015) *The Capitalist Unconscious*. London: Verso.
16 On mutative interpretation, but as engineered by the analyst, see Strachey, J. (1934) 'The Nature of the Therapeutic Action of Psycho-Analysis', *International Journal of Psycho-Analysis*, 15, pp. 127–159.
17 For a development of these questions, see Mandel, E. (1977) 'The Leninist Theory of Organisation', in R. Blackburn (ed.) *Revolution and Class Struggle: A Reader in Marxist Politics*. London: Fontana; Mandel, E. (2005) *Dictatorship of the Proletariat and Socialist Democracy*, www.marxists.org/archive/mandel/1985/dictprole/part1.htm.
18 On the 'half-said', see Lacan, J. (1987) 'Television', October, 40, pp. 7–50.
19 Freud, S. (1930) *Civilization and Its Discontents*, in S. Freud (1966–1974) *The Standard Edition of the Complete Psychological Works of Sigmund Freud* (translated by J. Strachey). London: Vintage, The Hogarth Press and the Institute of Psycho-Analysis, vol. XXI.
20 On the 'subject of science', see Lacan, J. (1965) 'Science and Truth', in J. Lacan (ed.) (2006) *Écrits: The First Complete Edition in English* (translated with notes by B. Fink in collaboration with H. Fink and R. Grigg). New York: Norton.
21 See Engels, F. (1883) *Dialectics of Nature*, www.marxists.org/archive/marx/works/download/EngelsDialectics_of_Nature_part.pdf and, for where this can lead under Stalinism, see Lecourt, D. (1976/1977) *Proletarian Science? The Case of Lysenko*. London: New Left Books.
22 On Marxism as the standpoint of the working class, see McCarney, J. (1990) *Social Theory and the Crisis of Marxism*. London: Verso.
23 On nationalism as a regression within Marxism, see Mandel, E. (1978) *From Stalinism to Eurocommunism: The Bitter Fruits of 'Socialism in One Country'*. London: New Left Books.
24 For the claim that it is possible to escape capitalism, see Bruno, P. op cit.
25 See Marx, K. (1867) *Capital: A Critique of Political Economy*, www.marxists.org/archive/marx/works/1867-c1/ (accessed 10 July 2018), and on the historical conditions of possibility for the phenomenon and critique, see Mandel, E. (1971) *The Formation of the Economic Thought of Karl Marx*. London: New Left Books.
26 On the historical status of psychoanalysis and its clinical context, see Dunker, C. (2010) *The Structure and Constitution of the Psychoanalytic Clinic: Negativity and Conflict in Contemporary Practice*. London: Karnac.
27 On contemporary capitalism and the rise of the service sector, see Mandel, E. (1974) *Late Capitalism*. London: New Left Books.
28 On new symptoms, see Redmond, J. (2014) *Ordinary Psychosis and the Body: A Contemporary Lacanian Approach*. London: Palgrave Macmillan.
29 This differs from the account offered by Tomšič, S., op cit.
30 For a conceptual and institutional history, see Roudinesco, E. (1990) *Jacques Lacan and Co.: A History of Psycho-Analysis in France 1925–1985*. London: Free Association Books.
31 This is the real that Žižek describes, drawing on Lévi-Strauss, but then indexing it, and class struggle, to sexual difference, in Žižek, S. (1999) *The Ticklish Subject: The Absent Centre of Political Ontology*. London: Verso.
32 See Freud, S. *Civilization and Its Discontents*, op cit., and on the translation from 'the unease inherent in culture', see Bettelheim, B. (1986) *Freud and Man's Soul*. Harmondsworth: Pelican.
33 On sexuation, see Lacan, J. (1975/1998) *On Feminine Sexuality, the Limits of Love and Knowledge, 1972–1973: Encore, The Seminar of Jacques Lacan, Book XX* (translated by B. Fink). New York: Norton; and for a critical Lacanian use of it to trace the transmission of sexual identity in the family, see Riggs, D. (2015) *Pink Herrings: Fantasy,*

Object Choice and Sexuation. London and New York: Routledge; Morris, B. (2020) *Sexual Difference, Abjection and Liminal Spaces: A Psychoanalytic Approach to the Abhorrence of the Feminine*. London and New York: Routledge.

34 On the Frankfurt School and feminist conceptions of 'second nature', see Young, R. M. (1992) 'Science, Ideology and Donna Haraway', *Science as Culture*, 15 (3), pp. 165–207.

35 For a Marxist account, see Geras, N. (1983) *Marx and Human Nature*. London: Verso.

36 For an account of Lacanian Discourse Analysis, see Pavón Cuéllar, D. (2010) *From the Conscious Interior to an Exterior Unconscious: Lacan, Discourse Analysis and Social Psychology*. London: Karnac.

37 For a feminist account of the linking of the 'personal and the political', see Rowbotham, S., Segal, L. and Wainwright, H. (2013) *Beyond the Fragments: Feminism and the Making of Socialism* (3rd ed.). Pontypool, Wales: Merlin.

38 For a wretched 'self-criticism' from within the French Communist Party, see Eight French Psychiatrists (Bonnafe, Follin, Kestemberg, Kestemberg, Lebovici, Le Guilland, Monnerot and Shentoub) (1949) 'Psychoanalysis: A Reactionary Ideology', *Marxism and Masses*, 2 (9), pp. 10–27.

39 For a non-Marxist but relevant social-anthropological critique of the induction into psychoanalysis as a worldview, see Gellner, E. (1985) *The Psychoanalytic Movement, or The Coming of Unreason*. London: Paladin.

Chapter 2

Capital's *Jouissance*

Society and Sexual Political Economy in Lacan's Marx

David Pavón-Cuéllar

Introduction

Society is often conceived as something superficial and deceptive that would disguise its own truth. Its truth would reside in its foundation, which would be something different from society, such as family in the most conservative ideologies, the State in Hegelian philosophy or simply the individuals who come together with shared interests in liberal individualistic thought. Marxism and psychoanalysis also unravel the fundamental truth of society beyond the apparent social unity: the former in the economy, in the forces and relations of production, in the classes and in their struggles; the latter in sexuality, in love and identification, in the Oedipal structure of the mass and in the primordial horde.

Society thus has a sexual foundation in psychoanalysis and an economic foundation in Marxism. The two foundations are obviously different. What is interesting is that Freud represented the functioning of sexuality in economic terms through what he called 'sexual' or 'libidinal economy'.

It is true that Freud's economics, at least at first glance, have absolutely nothing to do with those of Marx. The economic unit of Marxist theory is value, and not the amount of energy, as in Freudian theory. This is so because Freud's economy is based on thermodynamics while Marx's economy is political.

It is clear, then, that Marx and Freud do not understand economics in the same way. Nevertheless, the Freudian understanding of economic factors is often more akin to Marxist political economy than to thermodynamics. This is what happens, for example, when Freud associates the 'libidinal economy' with the satisfaction of needs and drives, with the performance of 'intellectual work' and with the purpose of 'fighting for happiness and moving away from misery'.[1] These all imply symbolic factors irreducible to the real of energy in thermodynamics.

In fact, in the Freudian theory of libidinal economy, energy appears not only as an objective amount of heat or physical power but also as the labour force of a subject who intervenes in a complex cultural process. This

DOI: 10.4324/9781003212072-3

becomes evident when Freud successively addresses dream-work, joke-work and mourning-work and considers in them the 'material' and its transformation, the 'psychic value' of what is transformed,[2] the 'technical resources' and the 'psychic products'[3] and the 'expenditure of time', not just 'energy'.[4] Including all these elements, Freud's work is not what work is in thermodynamics but what it is in political economy: a complex activity in which time is spent, energy is invested and technique is used for transforming a raw material and thus producing a value with which needs, drives or desires can be satisfied.

Although Freud was inspired by thermodynamics, his conception of the sexual economy corresponds more to the political economy. Lacan is right, therefore, when he categorically affirms that 'the economic references and configurations' of Marx were 'more suitable' than those 'coming from thermodynamics' for Freudian analysis.[5] Understanding this allows us to overcome the apparent discrepancy between Marxist and Freudian theories in their elucidation of the foundation of society by recognizing that both theories place this foundation in political economy, an economy whose sexual aspect is unavoidable, as I will demonstrate in the following pages.

This chapter will describe how Lacan incorporates sexuality in his reading of Marx's critical approach to political economy. I examine how this reading allows Lacan to consider the role of *enjoyment* (*jouissance*) in exchange and use values, reconceptualizing them as *enjoyment-value* and *enjoyment of value*. I also analyse how Lacan, resignifying psychoanalysis and not only Marxism, emphasizes the political character of Freud's sexual economy.

After examining how the relationship of the sexual and the social has been considered among various Freudian Marxist authors, I discuss some of Lacan's ideas about the sexual–economic foundation of society. I analyse the way in which these ideas, preceded by Jean Audard and based on Claude Lévi-Strauss, connect Marxist and Freudian concepts by founding society on the patriarchal exploitation of women. Patriarchy, according to Lacan, reaches not only its apogee in capitalist modernity but also its crisis, which manifests itself symptomatically through the discoveries of Marx and Freud.

I try to explain why Marxism and psychoanalysis constituted for Lacan the last strongholds of the subject, of use value and of knowledge in an increasingly automated capitalist system governed by exchange value and dominated by data and information. After glimpsing how capital monopolizes enjoyment in modern capitalist society, I will note that one must assume an enjoyment of capital to understand the Lacanian formulations in which exchange-value operates as enjoyment-value, use-value as enjoyment of value, and surplus-value as an expression of a *surplus-enjoyment* (*plus-de-jouir*), which is defined as the renunciation of enjoyment in the widespread discontent in culture. These formulations will help me to outline the way in which Lacan theorizes both Freud's sexual economy and the problem that concerns us now, that of sexuality as a principle of society.

The Problem of the Sexual as a Principle of the Social: Freudian Marxist Debates

The thesis of the social construction of sexuality is widely disseminated in gender studies and in the feminist movement. This spread has important political consequences. If women fight socially against patriarchal violence, it is because they assume that sexual problems, understood as gender problems, are fundamentally social and, therefore, must be dealt with in public spaces, on the street and in society. This idea, which today seems obvious, is not shared by Lacan.

Perhaps Lacan seems to us quite conservative when he considers that 'the problem posed by the sexual act is not social, since it is here where the principle of the social is constituted'.[6] For Lacan, society is founded on what is problematic about sexuality, not sexual problems being fundamentally social. More than a social construction of sexuality, what we have here is a sexual constitution of society. The social is the *explanandum*, while the sexual is the *explanans*.

The sexual explanation of the social is not exclusive to Lacanian theory but is a basic and central hypothesis of psychoanalysis. It was developed by Freud, mainly in *Totem and Taboo*[7] and in *Group Psychology and the Analysis of the Ego*.[8] Both works explain the existence of society and social groups by libidinal ties. These ties unite individuals, have an Oedipal structure and originate in the primordial horde.

Freudian social theory soon collided with other conceptions of society, including the Marxist one, which was especially influential in progressive environments more receptive to psychoanalysis. While Freud and his followers founded society on sexuality, Marxists founded it on the socio-economic base (i.e. the means and relations of production). This difference triggered passionate debates that reached their highest level of argumentation among Freudo-Marxists and other proponents of the Freudian left, who best knew the two disputed theses.

Henri de Man and Max Eastman were more inclined towards psychoanalysis. De Man challenged Marx's economism and replaced it with a psychologism in which all socio-economic life would obey psychological motivations, instincts and feelings.[9] Eastman rejected both psychology and the Marxist rationalist conception of economic rational determination, proposing instead the thesis of irrational determination by instincts and impulses.[10]

Similar to Eastman, Siegfried Bernfeld considered that the drives discovered by Freud underlay the economic forces elucidated by Marx; at the same time, he discarded the psychologism of those who tried to explain the economic sphere by inclinations and ideas. For Bernfeld, the psychological superstructure would rest on the economic infrastructure elucidated by Marxism, which in turn would rest on the base studied by psychoanalysis.[11]

By putting the drives at the base of the economic base, Bernfeld also engaged in a form of psychologization of the economic in the eyes of Wilhelm Reich, who preferred to draw a crucial distinction between rational behaviours (e.g. anti-capitalist revolutionary actions), economically determined and therefore explainable by Marxism, and irrational behaviours (e.g. those that submit to capitalism or support fascism), the explanation of which required recourse to psychoanalysis.[12]

The Reichian distinction was complicated by Attila József, who observed that all human beings act irrationally, obeying a consciousness that distorts and represses reality.[13] Similarly, in the Frankfurt School, irrationality operates within the very heart of rationality.[14] This is why József and those from Frankfurt think that we always need psychoanalytic sensitivity in addition to Marxism. Therefore, they agree with Jean Audard, who also concluded, like Eastman and Bernfeld, that irrationality underlies economic rationality.[15]

For Audard, Marxism needs psychoanalysis to be truly materialistic, i.e. to explain social life on the material basis of drives rather than the ideal scientific basis of productive technologies. The economic infrastructure unravelled by Marxism remains for Audard the basis of society, but it is divided into two superimposed levels, the deepest of which can only be studied by psychoanalysis. There is, therefore, no mutual exclusion between the Freudian and Marxist theories since we need both to probe the sexual–economic foundation of society. This is how Audard's Freudo-Marxism is justified.

From the Stallion to the Exchange of Women: Lévi-Strauss and the Emergence of Exchange-Value Understood as Value of Enjoyment

Lacan read Audard and was excited about his Freudo-Marxist conception. Many years later, Lacan elaborated on his own theoretical representation of the sexual–economic foundation of society, relying on the anthropology of Claude Lévi-Strauss, who in turn received the double influence of Marxism and psychoanalysis. Lévi-Strauss's *The Elemental Structures of Kinship* allowed Lacan, on the one hand, to confirm and reaffirm the Freudian idea of the sexual origin of society and, on the other hand, to understand this origin in the economic terms of Marxism.

Both the economic terms and the idea of the sexual origin are already found in the Levi-Straussian theory of generalized exchange.[16] This theory explains the existence of society as the union between patrilineal groups that must exchange women between them in order to ensure exogamy in each of them. Each group deprives itself of its sisters, mothers and other women, imposing the incest taboo, and gives them to other groups from whom it receives other women in return. In this exchange, women operate as sexual objects but also as economic objects – a kind of currency.

The exchange of women is at the origin not only of society but also of exchange value as understood in Marxist economic theory. The first object with an exchange value is the woman who is exchanged for another woman. The exchange value, for Lacan, is primarily a 'value of enjoyment', of 'possession', which supplants a use value (i.e. utility), like the value of the sex of a bull that fertilizes cows.[17]

The sex of the stallion gives way to the woman. After crossing this threshold of culture, which is also that of patriarchy, the woman becomes a phallic object. She starts working as a representation of the phallus, a detached object that is exchanged and circulated, a sex that is irretrievably detached from the stallion through castration, which is understood as the inaugural act of culture.

In the cultural world inaugurated by castration, man no longer has his essence in himself, but in woman – in the phallic object. This is how Lacan reinterprets an idea that is passed from Hegel and Feuerbach to the young Marx. This idea insists under different forms in the *Manuscripts* of 1844: (a) man 'becomes an object',[18] (b) objects present 'the essential forces of man'[19] and (c) the 'man's first object is man himself'.[20] When trying to 'give its true substance' to this idea, Lacan argues that the 'essence of man taken as an object' is, first of all, the woman with her 'phallic value' of exchange and enjoyment, a value that is later transferred to other objects that thus place themselves in the same place occupied by the woman – that of the use value of the sex of the stallion.[21]

It is not that the reproductive use value of the progenitor's sex is represented by the exchange value of the woman and other phallic objects. Rather, these objects, with their symbolic value, supplant and discard the real organ of the male. It is about castration, which – for Lacan – is also a symbolization that is directly linked to the process, widely studied in Marxism, by which exchange value progressively advances at the cost of the intrinsic use value of things.

The use value of the male sex mutates into the exchange value of the women who are exchanged between groups. After this mutation, as Lacan explains it, 'it is no longer the sexual organ of our bull – use-value – which will serve for this sort of circulation in which there is established the sexual order', but 'it is the woman, in so far as she herself has become on this occasion, the locus of transference of this value subtracted at the level of use value, in the form of object of *jouissance*'.[22] A symbolic cultural value, value of enjoyment and exchange, thus replaces the natural use-value of the stallion.

Women Who Pay the Price: Patriarchy and Exploitation in the Sexual–Economic Foundation of Society

The Lacanian idea of the mutation of the use of the stallion into the exchange of women is not only important because it explains the logical substitution of the real by the symbolic (i.e. substitution of the natural use-value by the cultural exchange-value). It is also important, as we have seen, because it tells us something about the hypothetical transition from matriarchy to patriarchy – a fundamental transition for Marxism but also, in some way, for psychoanalysis.

Let us remember how matriarchy appears in what Freud called the 'scientific myth' of the primordial horde.[23] In this mythical hypothesis, Freud certainly started from absolute paternal domination in the prehistoric horde, but he did not fail to recognize a matriarchal moment at the beginning of history, a moment after the dissolution of the horde and before the appearance of patriarchal society. First, in *Totem and Taboo*, Freud made Bachofen's 'maternal law institutions' coincide with the egalitarian organization based on 'homosexual feelings and activities' in which incest is forbidden and human civilization begins.[24] Then, in *Moses and Monotheism*, he identified a matriarchy in which women occupied 'a good part of the vacant plenipotence due to the elimination of the father' before being subjected again when 'maternal rights were relieved by a re-established patriarchal regime'.[25]

According to the Freudian myth, history and culture begin in matriarchy. The matriarchal moment is that of the dissolution of the primordial prehistoric horde and that of the establishment of the incest taboo. It is also a moment of brotherhood and equality, like the matriarchal phase of primitive communism for Marx and Engels.

Both Marxism and psychoanalysis accept the original reality of a horizontal, egalitarian and fraternal matriarchal society, which would have predated our patriarchal society marked by power, hierarchy, stratification and inequality. The essential link between verticality and patriarchy was also recognized by Freud, Marx and Engels. While Freud conceives the father as the primordial figure of power and authority, Marx and Engels discover a coincidence between the establishment of the patriarchal order and the emergence of private property (i.e. the division of society in classes and the beginning of appropriation and accumulation through the exploitation of man by man, which, by the way, was first an exploitation of woman by man).[26]

For the founders of Marxism and psychoanalysis, the essential link between patriarchy and vertical-oppressive relations is at the origin and foundation of our society. This sexual foundation is, for Marx and Engels, an economic foundation of appropriation, accumulation and exploitation, which has subsequently been emphasized by feminists of the Marxist tradition, such as Mariarosa Dalla Costa and Selma James,[27] as well as recently Silvia Federici.[28] The economic character of the sexual foundation of human society is also recognized in some way by Freud when he refers to the way in which human civilization absorbs a libido that 'withdraws a good part from women and from sexual life', up to the point that 'culture behaves with respect to sexuality like a class or group of people that has subjected another to exploit it'.[29]

It is very significant that both Freud and Marx put exploitation on the sexual–economic foundation of society. It should not be forgotten that this exploitation is inseparable from patriarchal oppression. Everything seems to start when men appropriate women and treat them as objects, enjoying them as their possession and exchanging them with each other. In these exchanges, as Lacan has well observed, 'it is the woman who pays the price'.[30] It is she who is exploited to enable the exchange on which society rests.

Social Decline of the Paternal Imago: Marxism and Psychoanalysis as Symptoms of the Crisis of Patriarchy

Before male domination and the exchange of women, there would be that mythical moment in which women would not have been simple objects of change and men would have acted as brothers, equitably sharing social goods with women and each other. It doesn't matter if all of this was a reality or part of a reality or just a myth. The important thing is that it can be conceived and thus, perhaps, motivate struggles against patriarchy and the inequality of class society.

Many of the great egalitarian and anti-patriarchal struggles of the 19th, 20th and 21st centuries have been inspired or at least influenced by Marxism. A good example is that of the Spartacus League with its historical expression in the Berlin commune of 1919 and with the famous leadership of Rosa Luxembourg, Karl Liebknecht and Clara Zetkin. This case was analysed by the psychoanalyst Paul Federn, who saw both a sign of the crisis of the father figure and the promise of an egalitarian, horizontal socialization, composed of subjects who would disagree with the Freudian representation of the human being as a horde animal.[31]

Just as Federn found in Spartacist Marxism a symptom of the historical fall of the figure of the father, so the young Lacan discovered this same symptom in psychoanalysis, interpreting it as an effect of the 'social decline of the paternal imago'.[32] This interpretation, carried out under the influence of Durkheim,[33] is quite justified by the castration complex, the universality of bisexuality and other Freudian formulas clearly unfavourable to the patriarchal conception of fatherhood and masculinity. If psychoanalysis represents a crisis of patriarchy, it is perhaps mainly for the same reason that Marxism also represents that crisis: because both, as we have appreciated, probe the sexual–economic foundation of patriarchal society and conceive a matriarchal alternative, projecting it into the mythical origin of civilization.

Perhaps Marxism and psychoanalysis contribute to deepening the crisis of patriarchy, but they are basically symptoms, expressions and effects – not causes – of the crisis. The aetiology of this crisis is more difficult to establish. What is certain is that it has to do with modernity and specifically with capitalism, which have meant both the culmination and the crisis of patriarchy.

The father figure is both undermined and reinforced by modern capitalist society. As Ian Parker has so well pointed out, 'the reorganization of the nuclear family under capitalism installs the father as master in the house at the same time that it takes away his power'.[34] These two opposite faces of the father, as castrating and castrated, have been conceptualized in psychoanalysis and are manifested in various typical phenomena of the modern capitalist world.

Capital directly strengthens patriarchy by defending family private property dominated by the father, by overrating the production of wealth at the cost of the reproduction of life, by ignoring or devaluing the domestic-reproductive work generally performed by women, by overvaluing lucrative-productive work carried out predominantly by men and by putting exchange value over use value. The patriarchal order is also indirectly benefited by capitalism that accentuates oppressive relationships, uses repressive governmental functions, encourages discipline and obedience and contributes to appropriation, accumulation, inequality, hierarchical verticality and various forms of power concentration. At the same time, capitalism weakens patriarchy by liberating women in some way – liberating them from men in order to submit them to capital and to exploit them as labour and consumption power. In this situation, as in many others, the capitalist system undermines and erodes the patriarchal order because it imposes the power of capital over any other, subverts any authority and only strengthens the father to put itself in his place, subjugating and humiliating him and making him publicize and sell himself as a commodity.

Capitalism prevents men from retaining the traditional patriarchal privilege of enjoyment, possession, exchange and exploitation of women. Now, in the modern capitalist patriarchal society, it is no longer man but rather capital itself that enjoys all subjects, possessing them to exchange them as simple commodities and to exploit their lives as labour power or as purchasing power. This is how capitalism provokes the crisis of patriarchy, transmuting the patriarchal phallic *jouissance* – that of possession for possession – into a *jouissance* of capital.

Capital That Works Alone: The Plunder of Knowledge and the Automation of Capitalism

If the capitalist system has less and less need of men with their patriarchal dignity, it is for the same reason that it has less and less need of human beings with their heritage of civilization. Humanity is increasingly unnecessary for capitalism to enjoy humanity, which was already recognized by Marx when observing the automation of the production process with the relentless advance of constant capital (i.e. technology) at the cost of variable capital (i.e. labour power). Workers lose importance as technological advances allow more and more functions of human beings to be fulfilled by the capitalist automaton, which tends to be self-sufficient.

The automation of capitalism once raised the hope that human beings could finally free themselves from manual labour, leaving it to automatic devices, and thereby dedicate themselves exclusively to intellectual work (e.g. making decisions and organizing processes), which would allow them to dominate the great capitalist machinery just as they dominate any machine. The utopian illusions of the post-industrial society were those of a final triumph of humanity over the enjoyment of capital in a society without exploited proletarians, a society dominated by white-collar workers, pure chief engineers and technocrats using their knowledge as power to exploit the capitalist machinery.[35] What was not foreseen was that this machinery, ironically thanks to technological advances, would also be capable of carrying out increasingly complex intellectual work and that it could thus continue to sustain its enjoyment, proletarianizing human beings, reducing them to appendages of the machine – perhaps no longer as a manual labour force but, instead, as a kind of intellectual labour force.

In fact, when we look more closely at the brain work we do today, we realize that it is not really intellectual work but, rather, a kind of intellectually manual work. It is a simple manipulation of information and data that are generated automatically and that allow us to carry out certain operations on a scheduled basis. The capitalist automaton programs what we do, guides our decisions and produces what we manipulate. We only perform the tasks that we must perform. We do not create anything, nor do we express ourselves in what we do. Our work is as alien to us as that of the proletarians in the factory is alien to them. Both works are alienated; they belong not to the person who performs them but to the Other – to capitalism.

It is capital that enjoys what the manual and intellectual proletarians do. Since they know absolutely nothing about what they do, capitalism should have some knowledge that clarifies everything for us. However, being nothing more than an economic system of production, capital cannot know anything. Instead of knowledge, capitalism contains only data and information. This is all that remains of the knowledge whose history was reconstructed by Marx and Lacan.

Knowledge belonged first to slaves, serfs, servants and artisans – to traditional workers, whose work was simultaneously manual and intellectual. Little by little, as manual and intellectual work diverged, the former workers were proletarianized and turned into exclusively manual workers, having been plundered of their knowledge that was transferred to the masters. As Lacan conceives it, this change of position of knowledge consisted of putting oneself in the epistemologically sanctioned 'good position' of the master and in converting the knowledge of a slave into the 'knowledge of a master', which was the work of philosophy and is at the origin of modern science.[36] The result is the figure of the scientist, the engineer, the professional and the intellectual worker in general, who monopolizes knowledge, which originally belonged to the artisans and other workers, but which later dissociated itself from them and finally served to enjoy them, to possess them and to exploit them as proletarians.

After the manual workers were robbed of their knowledge, it was the turn of the intellectual workers, who also had to give up their knowledge to computers and other machines of the capitalist automaton. Knowledge has thus materialized into technology, ceasing to be what it was (i.e. knowledge) to become designs, hardware and software, programs and instructions, data and information. This is what proletarianized intellectual workers manipulate, without knowing exactly what they are doing, when their intellectual labour force is exploited by the capitalist system. It is thus that the capital, the modern master of the masters, has ended up monopolizing the enjoyment that was first of the slaves and then of their masters.

Neither Commerce with Marx nor Defraud with Freud: Strongholds of Use Value in a World Governed by Exchange Value

Capitalism exploits the intellectual work carried out with the technology of the 'social brain', the cultural heritage of human civilization, and individual brains, connected to the capitalist automaton as in the film *Matrix*. It is with this intellectual labour power that capital thinks as a computer thinks. This thought is no longer knowledge, since knowledge implies an experience and existence of a subject.

Instead of knowing, the capitalist system computes and calculates. It is an endless exchange of information devoid of a value inherent to it. Its only value is the exchange value, extrinsic and quantitative, which continues to gain ground at the cost of use value, intrinsic and qualitative.

Use value must take refuge somewhere. It takes refuge in what remains of true knowledge, that which cannot be exchanged and only 'enters with hard experiences', as Lacan says. This non-exchangeable knowledge is what we still find bequeathed to us by Marx and Freud. As Lacan says, 'with Marx's knowledge of politics one cannot do *comarx* (*commarxe*), no more than one can, with Freud's knowledge, defraud'.[37]

We cannot do commerce or defraud with what Marx and Freud teach us, with their heritage of non-negotiable, non-transferable and unsaleable knowledge, which is an exception in our world where everything is bought, circulated and exchanged. In the great market inaugurated by the exchange of women, Marxism and psychoanalysis also constitute symptoms of the crisis of patriarchy because they open spaces freed from the patriarchal logic of phallic *jouissance*, of possession and exchange. It must be well understood that this logic underlies the capitalist system and governs all its operations.

In capitalism, everything becomes the object of capital's enjoyment, of appropriation and accumulation, exploitation and business, fraud and commerce. Everything thus becomes an object of exchange, a commodity with an exchange value represented by money. We can pay for everything, including substitutes for knowledge (e.g. data, information, training, university degrees and even books on Marx and Freud) as well as courses in psychoanalysis or psychoanalytic treatments. No matter how much we pay, however, it is not likely that, by doing fraud and commerce, we will be able to buy the knowledge that Freud and Marx offer us in the clinic and in politics, respectively.

The knowledge offered by Marx and Freud can only be obtained when subjects commit themselves – when they put their own lives, their own bodies, in analysis and militancy, on the couch and in the street. This does not mean a relapse into empiricism, as certain formalist readings of Lacan have supposed, since it is not only about subjective experience; it is about subjects themselves, their existence, their vital and corporal materiality, beyond any experience. Marxism and psychoanalysis, especially Lacanian psychoanalysis, are certainly incompatible with empiricism, but not with materialism.

We have to give ourselves materially, and not only experience ourselves, to reach the enigmatic knowledge in which it seems that class consciousness is acquired and the unconscious becomes conscious. It is as if our material involvement allowed us to reach a consciousness that would be the necessary condition of any use value of knowledge for us. Of course, it is not exactly this, but rather a question of knowledge that is not necessarily conscious, although this does not mean that it lacks a unique use value for the subject who acquires it – a singular intrinsic value that cannot be obtained in exchange.

Use value is advocated by both Marxism and psychoanalysis, which do not focus only on exchange value as has been imagined in other formalist interpretations of Lacanian theory. The truth is that Lacan saw very well the centrality of use value in the traditions founded by Marx and Freud. Marxism and psychoanalysis, as Lacan conceives them, represent strongholds of a use value that is unaffordable through exchange value in a capitalist system in which everything seems to have an exchange value.

Renunciation of Capital's *Jouissance*: Enjoyment Value and Enjoyment of Value

We know that exchange value, as Lacan has shown, is a value of possession, of *jouissance* that tends to be that of capital in the capitalist system. In this system, the enjoyment of capital, clearly manifested in the possession for the possession of capitalist accumulation, is what gives all commodities their exchange value and what ultimately drives not only their exchange, purchase and sale but also their production. As Marx well demonstrated, everything is produced and circulates in capitalism only for capital to enjoy, to accumulate – to be more and more the same as it is at the cost of everything else.

The things produced and exchanged in capitalism also have a use value, of course. They feed us, dress us, shelter us and entertain us. If these things have been produced and sold, however, it is generally to produce a surplus value so that more capital is possessed. It is for the enjoyment of capital that we are made to pay the price that expresses the value of capital's enjoyment. This value is the exchange value of the things we buy.

Maybe we buy things because they have a use value for our lives, but this value is not what makes them exist. If they exist for a use value, it is the lucrative use value they have for the accumulation of capital and for its enjoyment. It is the same with the lucrative use value of human life, exploited as capital's labour force. If capitalism allows this life to reproduce itself, it is just for its usefulness for the enjoyment of capital. It is thus also, indirectly, how capital enjoys the use value that things have for our lives, thus confirming, in all cases, that the use value, as Lacan says, is 'something that is enjoyed'.[38]

Capital's enjoyment includes both the use value (i.e. the value it enjoys) and the exchange value (i.e. the value of its enjoyment). All value is subsumed in the capital and subordinated to its enjoyment. The interesting thing here is that capital cannot enjoy in the strict sense since it is nothing more than an impersonal, inert and insensitive process. This process needs the subjects to enjoy through them, but the enjoyment is still of capital.

It is capital that enjoys through subjects who only know *jouissance* negatively as dispossession or 'renunciation of *jouissance*'.[39] Even the capitalist must renounce the enjoyment that is fundamentally of capital and not of the person who personifies it. It is through this renunciation that dispassionate, cold and calculating capitalists distinguish themselves, according to Marx, from the figures of hoarders and misers who enjoy their wealth.[40] While hoarders enjoy what they possess, capitalists must renounce the enjoyment of which they are a part: the enjoyment of capital.[41]

Discontent as Renunciation: Culture in Capitalist Modernity

Possessed by what they think they possess, efficient capitalists are like other subjects who adequately play their role in capitalism. Everyone has to renounce the enjoyment that is increasingly monopolized by capital. Hence, we all suffer from the enjoyment that is not ours. It is also because of this that, according to Lacan, we all are proletarians suffering from 'the only social symptom', that of our 'proletarian' condition.[42] Proletarianization affects all of us in capitalist societies because we all work in one way or another for capital; possessed and exploited by it, we all have to renounce its enjoyment.

Of course, the renunciation of enjoyment is not exclusive to capitalist modern society. Previous societies were also structured by symbolic systems that imposed a certain renunciation. The Other has always enjoyed at the expense of the subjects, but capitalism was necessary for both the enjoyment of the Other and the renunciation of it to be accentuated to the point of provoking symptoms such as those manifested in Marxism and psychoanalysis.

Both Marx's proletarians and Freud's hysterics and neurotics suffer from the same enjoyment of the Other that all other subjects in modern society suffer. Just as we are all proletarianized, so we are all hystericized and neuroticized. This is something that has been very well understood in psychoanalysis, especially in Marxist psychoanalysis, which is very significant. Attila József, for example, has already diagnosed the 'disease' that we all suffer from,[43] while Norman O. Brown defined man as a 'neurotic' or 'discontented animal'.[44]

According to Lacan, 'discontent' in Freud's culture corresponds precisely to the 'renunciation of *jouissance*'.[45] It should not be forgotten that Freud himself has already put the 'renunciation of instinctual satisfaction' at the very foundation of human culture.[46] If humanity is condemned to discontent, it is because culture is based on enjoyment and the renunciation of enjoyment, on the satisfaction of the death drive and on the renunciation of this satisfaction. All this is very well explained by Freud.[47]

What is clarified thanks to Marx is that subjects must renounce the satisfaction of the death drive to leave this satisfaction to capital so that capital monopolizes deadly enjoyment, transmuting everything that is alive into what is dead, thus into more and more inert capital. The enjoyment of capital, as we have seen, is the correlate of the subject's renunciation of this enjoyment. It is also for this reason that Lacan understands this renunciation of *jouissance* as a surplus-enjoyment (*plus-de-jouir*) equivalent to Marx's surplus-value.

Surplus-Enjoyment in Surplus-Value: Difference Between Your Money and Your Life

Surplus-value is the only form in which the enjoyment of capital can appear in the capitalist economic sphere. Capital cannot enjoy itself, but only value itself, which produces a surplus-value. This production of a supplement of value is the enjoyment of capital, which is experienced through the subjects as a renunciation of enjoyment – as a surplus-enjoyment that is lost so that capital gains its surplus-value.

Lacan shows how surplus-value is the form of surplus-enjoyment in the 'absolutization of the market' that is characteristic of capitalism.[48] As described in Marx, this absolutization makes all things and people intervene as commodities that are exchanged for each other according to their exchange value. Generalized exchange cannot include the enjoyment, which cannot circulate, but does include its exchange value, the enjoyment-value, the value of the renunciation of enjoyment and the value of surplus-enjoyment, which is the surplus-value.

Marx must have calculated surplus-value to describe the capitalist absolutized market, but he was always aware that he was referring to surplus-enjoyment – to something incalculable that underlay surplus-value. Marx always understood that surplus-value not only resulted from the quantitative difference between two commensurable values, the lower exchange-value and the higher use-value of labour power, but also designated the qualitative difference between money and life, between the negligible value of the enjoyment of work and the enjoyment of its value for capital, between the value that workers earn and the enjoyment they must renounce. What Marx always understood, in other words, is that surplus-value was the surplus-enjoyment that capital gained and that the subject lost when they exchanged the former's money for the existence of the latter.

Marx always knew that surplus-value is the product of the exchange between something real and something purely symbolic, between the existence of the worker and the value of capital, between something living and something dead. What is gained is the dead – the value – in exchange for the living, thus satisfying the death drive of capital. This deadly enjoyment of capital, of the 'vampire' who lives by 'sucking living labour', was located by Marx at the very origin of surplus-value.[49]

It was at the very threshold of the production of a supplement of value that Marx glimpsed what Lacan later called 'surplus-enjoyment'. This can be verified in the unpublished chapter VI of *Capital*, when Marx describes the starting point of the entire capitalist process: the 'exchange of less objectified labour for more living labour'.[50] The exchange is not only between more and less value, as in surplus-value, but between two different labours, one alive and the other objectified. In exchange for a dead object, labourers give the enjoyment of their life to capital.

Surplus-Value and Surplus-Enjoyment: Enjoyment of Capital and Suffering of the Subject, Wealth and Poverty, Development and Underdevelopment

Glimpsing the surplus-enjoyment and not reducing everything to the calculation of values from which surplus-value results, Marx does not make the mistake of offering a supposed absolute knowledge to describe the functioning of the absolutized market. What interests him in this market is not the patent generalized exchange governed by exchange-value, but the latent – what must be lost for this exchange to be possible. It is in this that Marx differs from the philosopher and the economist (i.e. from Hegel and Smith or Ricardo), who in one way or another did aspire to absolutize knowledge at the expense of knowledge itself.

Knowledge is lost in its absolutization because it omits what constitutes it internally, the involvement of subjects and their lives, their bodies and their surplus-enjoyment. As Lacan explains, this 'price' of 'renunciation of *jouissance*', as considered by Marx, is what makes knowledge exist without being absolute like absolutized capitalism.[51] Certainly, as Lacan also saw, there is a 'fierceness of Marx in castrating himself' that reveals an aspiration to 'absolute knowledge', which is displayed in *Capital* and in the attempt to 'calculate' surplus-value.[52] However, as the capitalist's laugh shows, Marx knows that the important thing is elsewhere. This is why, on the one hand, his economic calculations try to apprehend something incalculable, as Lacan demonstrated, and, on the other hand, his concepts of value and surplus-value 'designate non-economic realities that are not measurable, not quantifiable', as Althusser showed.[53]

Thanks to his consideration of the unquantifiable and immeasurable surplus-enjoyment, what Marx offers us is true knowledge that can represent today, like Freud's inheritance, a redoubt of knowledge in the midst of the circulation of data and information. This generalized exchange seems to totally dispense with subjects by operating automatically through interconnected computers all over the world, while Marxism and psychoanalysis involve subjects who struggle and who analyse themselves, who make their own history, who renounce enjoyment and suffer the surplus-enjoyment. This is how the Marxist and Freudian heritages allow us to know something about the production conditions of our world, about its truth that is manifested symptomatically in hysterical subversion or in the proletarian revolution and that lays in the surplus-enjoyment and not in the surplus-value, in the suffering of the subjects and not in the enjoyment of capital, in misery and not in wealth and in underdevelopment and not in development.

Lacan stated categorically that 'development leads to underdevelopment'.[54] We can even say that development presupposes underdevelopment as its condition of possibility and as its condition of production, as we saw that surplus-enjoyment is presupposed in surplus-value. Rosa Luxembourg understood this, and that is why she found the condition of development outside of development and capitalist accumulation.[55] The same was confirmed by Dependency and Third World Theories, which understood that underdevelopment is the foundation of development and that Africa must be underdeveloped to develop Europe.[56]

Conclusion

Developed capitalism cannot be constituted only by capital's *jouissance*; it requires a place for the subject, for knowledge and for the renunciation of enjoyment. This place is that of underdevelopment, but also that of Marxism, psychoanalysis and the other spaces in which something can be known about discontent in culture, about the surplus-enjoyment, understood as the subjective correlate of the surplus-value in which the enjoyment of capital lies.

Elucidating the sexual–economic foundation of modern capitalist society, Lacan has allowed us to infer the capital's *jouissance* from his re-politicization of Freud's sexual economy and his re-sexualization of Marx's political economy. Both operations help us to glimpse a Lacanian economic-sexual theory centred on the following reformulations: (a) possession as enjoyment of the Other monopolized by capital in capitalism, (b) exchange-value as value of that enjoyment in generalized exchange, (c) use-value as enjoyment of the value for the capital that possesses and exploits it and (d) surplus-value as surplus-enjoyment, as surplus of enjoyment for the capital that can only be enjoyed through the subject's renunciation of enjoyment. Finally, there is discontent in culture because no one can enjoy except someone who is not someone, but something that needs the subjects to enjoy: the condensation of the symbolic in the vampire of capital, who satisfies the death drive through the subjects by exploiting them, by enjoying them, by devouring their life to produce dead money.

While capital enjoys through the subjects, they suffer its enjoyment, the renunciation of enjoyment and the exploitation of their lives for the enjoyment of capital. This suffering is the price that subjects must pay to know something in Marxism and psychoanalysis. What they know is what the proletarians taught Marx and what the hysterics taught Freud. It is what underlies the transactions in the market, the circulation of data and information and the generalized exchange based on the exchange values of goods. It is the surplus-enjoyment in the surplus-value. It is the enjoyment of the Other, of capital, that gives its value to exchange-value. It is the enjoyment of the value of everything – the use value of everything – monopolized by capital.

Notes

1 Sigmund Freud, El malestar en la cultura (1929), in *Obras completas XIV*, Buenos Aires, Amorrortu, 1998, pp. 78–79.
2 Freud, La interpretación de los sueños (primera parte) (1900), in *Obras completas IV*, Buenos Aires, Amorrortu, 1998, pp. 285–343.
3 Freud, El chiste y su relación con lo inconsciente (1905), in *Obras completas VIII*, Buenos Aires, Amorrortu, 1998, pp. 83–84.
4 Freud, Duelo y melancolía (1917), in *Obras completas XIV*, Buenos Aires, Amorrortu, 1998, pp. 242–243.
5 Jacques Lacan, *Le séminaire, Livre XVI, D'un Autre à l'autre* (1968–1969), Paris, Seuil, 2006, p. 21.
6 J. Lacan, *Le séminaire, Livre XV, La logique du fantasme*, unpublished, April 12, 1967.
7 Freud, Tótem y Tabú (1913), in *Obras completas XIII*, Buenos Aires, Amorrortu, 1998.

8 Freud, Psicología de las masas y análisis del yo (1921), in *Obras completas XVIII*, Buenos Aires, Amorrortu, 1998.
9 Henri De Man, *Au-delà du marxisme* (1926), Paris, Seuil, 1974.
10 Max Eastman, *Marx and Lenin: The Science of Revolution* (1927), New York, Albert and Charles Boni.
11 Siegfried Bernfeld, *Sisyphus or The Limits of Education* (1925), Berkeley, University of California Press, 1973.
12 Wilhelm Reich, *Materialismo dialéctico y psicoanálisis* (1934), Mexico City, Siglo XXI, 1989.
13 Attila József, Hegel, Marx, Freud (1934), *Action Poétique* 49 (1972), 68–75.
14 E. g. Max Horkheimer, Historia y psicología (1932), in *Teoría crítica*, Buenos Aires: Amorrortu, 2008.
15 Jean Audard, Du caractère matérialiste de la psychanalyse (1933), *Littoral* 27/28 (1989), 199–208.
16 Claude Lévi-Strauss, *Les structures élémentaires de la parenté* (1949), Paris, Mouton, 1967.
17 J. Lacan, *Le séminaire, Livre XV, La logique du fantasme,* unpublished, April 12, 1967.
18 Karl Marx, *Manuscritos, economía y filosofía* (1844), Madrid, Alianza, 1997, p. 149.
19 Ibid., p. 151.
20 Ibid., p. 153.
21 J. Lacan, *Le séminaire, Livre XV, La logique du fantasme,* unpublished, April 12, 1967.
22 Ibid.
23 Freud, Psicología de las masas y análisis del yo (1921), en *Obras completas XVIII*, Buenos Aires, Amorrortu, 1997, p. 128.
24 Freud, Tótem y tabú (1913), in *Obras completas XIII*, Buenos Aires, Amorrortu, 1997, p. 146.
25 Freud, Moisés y la religión monoteísta (1939), en *Obras completas XXIII*, Buenos Aires, Amorrortu, 1997, p. 79.
26 Marx, *Los apuntes etnológicos de Karl Marx* (1882), Madrid, Siglo XXI & Pablo Iglesias, 1988. Friedrich Engels, *El origen de la familia, de la propiedad privada y del Estado* (1884), Mexico City, Colofón, 2011.
27 E.g. Mariarosa Dalla Costa y Selma James, The power of women and the subversion of the community, in Rediker, M., & Lopez, N. (Eds), *Sex, Race and Class, the Perspective of Winning: A Selection of Writings 1952–2011.* Oakland, Selma James, 1972.
28 Silvia Federici, *El patriarcado del salario, críticas feministas al marxismo*, Madrid y Ciudad de México, Traficantes de Sueños y Universidad Autónoma de la Ciudad de México, 2018.
29 Freud, El malestar en la cultura (1929), en *Obras completas XXIII*, Buenos Aires, Amorrortu, 1997, pp. 101–102.
30 J. Lacan, *Le séminaire, Livre XV, La logique du fantasme*, unpublished, April 12, 1967.
31 Paul Federn, De la psychologie de la révolution: la société sans père (1919), *Essaim 5* (2000), 166
32 Jacques Lacan, Les complexes familiaux dans la formation de l'individu (1938), en *Autres écrits*, París, Seuil, 2001, p. 61
33 See Markos Zafiropoulos, Le déclin du père, *Topique*, 84(3) (2003), 161–171.
34 Ian Parker, *Lacanian Psychoanalysis. Revolutions in Subjectivity* (2011), London, Routledge, p. 56.
35 E.g. Daniel Bell, *The Coming of Post-Industrial Society: A Venture in Social Forecasting* (1973), New York, Basic Books.
36 J. Lacan, *Le séminaire, Livre XVII, L'envers de la psychanalyse* (1991), Paris, Seuil, pp. 20–23.
37 J. Lacan, *Le séminaire, Livre XX, Encore* (1999), Paris, Seuil (poche), pp. 124–125.

38 J. Lacan, Conférence au Musée de la science et de la technique de Milan, in *Lacan in Italia 1953–1978* (1978), Milan, La Salamandra, p. 69.
39 J. Lacan, *Le séminaire, Livre XVI, D'un Autre à l'autre* (1968–1969), Paris, Seuil, 2006, p. 39.
40 Marx, *El Capital* (1867), Mexico City, FCE, 2008, pp. 88–92.
41 See Samo Tomsic, *The Capitalist Unconscious: Marx and Lacan* (2016), London, Verso, pp. 68–69.
42 Lacan, La troisième, intervention au Congrès de Rome, in *Lettres de l'École freudienne*, 16, 1975, p. 187.
43 József, Hegel, Marx, Freud (1934), *Action Poétique* 49 (1972), p. 75.
44 Norman O. Brown, *Life Against Death. The Psychoanalytical Meaning of History* (1959), Middletown, Wesleyan University Press, 1985, p. 90.
45 Lacan, *Le séminaire, Livre XVI, D'un Autre à l'autre* (1968–1969), op. cit., pp. 40–41.
46 Freud, El porvenir de una ilusión (1927), in *Obras completas XIV*, Buenos Aires, Amorrortu, 1998, p. 7.
47 Freud, El malestar en la cultura (1929), op. cit., pp. 100–104.
48 Lacan, *Le séminaire, Livre XVI, D'un Autre à l'autre* (1968–1969), op. cit., p. 37.
49 Marx, *El Capital* (1867), Mexico City, FCE, 2008, p. 179.
50 Marx, *El Capital. Libro I. Capítulo VI (inédito). Resultados del proceso inmediato de producción* (1866), Mexico City, Siglo XXI, 2009, p. 42.
51 Lacan, *Le séminaire, Livre XVI, D'un Autre à l'autre* (1968–1969), op. cit., 40–41.
52 Lacan, *Le séminaire, Livre XVII, L'envers de la psychanalyse* (1969–1970), op. cit., pp. 123–124.
53 Althusser, L'objet du *Capital*, in *Lire Le Capital* (1965), Paris, PUF, 1996, pp. 258–259.
54 Lacan, *Le séminaire, Livre XVIII, D'un discours qui ne serait pas du semblant* (1970–1971), Paris, Seuil, 2007, p. 51.
55 Rosa Luxemburgo, *La acumulación del capital* (1913), La Plata, Terramar, 2007.
56 See Walter Rodney, *How Europe Underdeveloped Africa* (1972), London, Verso Trade, 2018.

Chapter 3

Can We Decolonize Lacan? Indigenous Origins of the Split Subject

Clint Burnham

What does it mean to ask if we can decolonize Lacan? Is this to argue we should think about psychoanalysis in the context of decolonial thought, or does it mean to search through the Lacanian archive and root out either problematic utterances *or* points of possible conjunction? Does it mean to ask if we *ought* to decolonize Lacan, or does it mean to ask if it is possible to decolonize Lacan? Does it mean to ask who is the "we" in the sentence – clinicians or theorists, colonized peoples or settlers? Perhaps asking "can we decolonize Lacan" means not so much providing an *answer* but, in a reflexive or "meta" fashion, speculating on what it means to ask that question, why we are asking it now, and how or whether decolonizing Lacan also means Lacanizing or psychoanalyzing the decolonial struggle. In what follows, I propose that decolonizing Lacan entails, first, exploring how to think psychoanalytically about the geospatial (from Freud's narcissism of small differences to Said's "travelling theory") in terms of the "decolonial turn" that draws on Fanon's theoretical readings as well as Enrique Dussell and Walter Mignolo's critiques of modernity. How, for instance, are we to *read* Lacan in relation to Algeria, or to bring Freud's notion of the neighbor to bear on Indigenous or Black feminist thought? To answer this requires a spatial logic that abjures the holistic or substantial for a *Spaltung* or splitting of the subject, which theory, in Lacan, both derives from Kwakwākā'wakw or Pacific Northwest Coast masks and traditions, and in turn, via such formalizations as the L-schema, suggests a scaling up and back to contemporary Indigenous theorizations as found in the Haida-Québecois artist Raymond Boisjoly.

Put in a more concise way, this chapter reads Lacan in terms of some of the spatial questions that have been developed in decolonial theory, moving from spatiality thought at a geopolitical level down to that of the subject (and back again). Anne Anlin Cheng argued in 2000 that the politics of race has always spoken in the language of psychoanalysis, pointing out that "*intrasubjectivity exists as a form of intersubjectivity* and that *intersubjectivity often speaks in the voice of intrasubjectivity*" (28). So, in exploring some global questions of decolonizing psychoanalysis, I mean *global* in two senses: both the spatial geographies of Lacanian and decolonial theory, and the master

DOI: 10.4324/9781003212072-4

signifiers or concepts of those theories, how they can be read together. For just as we can think of *geographies of decolonization*, as a shift away from the historical narrative of post–World War II or post–Cold War decolonial struggles, so too we can think of the *geographies* of Lacanian thought but also the spatial dimensions of that thought itself, such as when Derrida (1998), in his contribution to *Psychoanalysis and Race*, engages in a "geopsychoanalysis" by way of critiquing the IPA's Euro-provincialism. This is what Ranjana Khanna (2003), commenting on Derrida but drawing on Heidegger and Spivak, calls "worlding psychoanalysis," or determining, through a critical reading practice, not only how psychoanalysis comes into being with others as its underside, "primitive beings against which the modern European self, in need of psychoanalysis, was situated," but also the conundrum that such a provincialization or parochialism of European psychoanalysis (she also draws on Dipesh Chakrabarty) "does not explain adequately why [psychoanalysis] has persisted, or indeed why it was used by theorists of decolonization" (2–3, 100). These geographies of psychoanalysis mean that when we turn to the trajectories and genealogies of Lacanian concepts – here, the split subject – we find what Cedric Robinson (1993, 86) has called "radical anticipations" of Lacan among *les damnées* which in turn incite a rethinking of the spatial.

Given the topic of this chapter – the split subject, the mask, and the decolonial – it would be remiss not to discuss Fanon's *Black Skin, White Masks.* I will restrict myself to the question of a split, as it were, in the reception of *BSWM* at two historical junctures: first, the post-structuralist hegemony of the 1980s and 1990s (epitomized in the discussions by Bhabha [1986, 1996], Gates [1991], Robinson [1993], Parry [1987], and Hall [1996]); and second, the decolonial debates of the 2010s (Zabala [2012], Dabashi [2013/2016], Mignolo [2013], Žižek [2016], Beshara [2018]). In that first moment, we very much see a willingness, on the part of Bhabha and Hall in particular, to read Fanon through a Lacanian lens (albeit not "our Lacan," as I said to Gautam Basu Thakur in an email – not the Lacan that has been periodized into early [Imaginary], middle [Symbolic] and late [Real] Lacan, but the Lacan of the 1980s reception, of the mirror stage and the look). For this reading, Bhabha especially (and his 1986 introduction to the Pluto edition of *BSWM* in particular) is excoriated by Robinson, Parry, and Gates, because of his recruiting Fanon to the post-structuralist discourses ("premature post-structuralism," as Parry puts it [1987, 31], "turning Fanon into *le Lacan noir*," as Gates says [1991, 462]) of anti-foundationalism, refusal of an unproblematic native voice, and, what is perhaps most symptomatic in Robinson's *foreclosure* of Bhabha, Fanon's analysis of bourgeois intellectuals' romanticization of the colonized – the "black abyss" (Fanon, 1986, 7; Robinson, 1993, 80). But Robinson is also critical of any attempt to read Fanon as a psychoanalyst, and so when Gates (1991) compares Freudian "analysis interminable" to Fanonian "decolonization interminable" (466), for Robinson this "compounds his negligence of Fanon, erases the contradictions and radical anticipations in Fanon . . . a metaphorical displacement of colonialist oppression by a therapeutic paradigm" (86). The predictable aversion, in Marxism, to psychoanalysis qua the "therapeutic" should not distract us, however, from Robinson's perspicacious remarks on Fanon's "contradictions and radical *anticipations*," which last we can see Robinson already formulating in his discussion, in *Black Marxism*, of the "strikes" (which is to say, desertion) of 100,000 poor whites from Confederate armies and half a million slaves from plantations as anticipating a revolution fifty years later: "it was the same pattern, indeed, which came to fruition in Russia" (2000, 271).[1]

Like my discussion, below, of how NWC Indigenous masks anticipate the Lacanian split subject, the Bhabha/Robinson debate anticipates the Mignolo/Žižek debate of the past decade. Now the argument is over whether European critics – on the basis of their geographic origin – should be read in the Global South: Dabashi takes issue with Zabala's list of European philosophers (including Žižek), and then Mignolo, citing Sartre, says "listen, pay attention. Fanon is no longer talking to us [that is, to Europeans]" (2013, n.p.). But this move of Mignolo's is rhetorically complex, to say the least, and not only for how he bases his argument that the South need not listen to the West on a thinker, Fanon, who evidently was very much drawing on such European thinkers as Hegel, Lacan, and Mannoni. The split, then, in 1980s and 1990s readings of Fanon – on whether he was a revolutionary or a post-structuralist – has been transformed into the question of a global split: spatiality scaled up from the subject to decolonial geographies.[2]

And so, while the engagement of psychoanalysis and race/decolonization goes back decades (see, in addition to Cheng, Khanna, and Derrida, Edward Said [2003], Kalpana Seshadri-Crooks [2000]), much work remains in two key areas. First, we need a reading of psychoanalysis, qua its canonical texts but also a genealogy of its concepts, in terms of both its colonial conditions (as Said [2003], Jacqueline Rose [1996], and Dušan Bjelić [2016] essay for Freud) and its racialized or colonizing tropologies and significations (as Ian Almond [2012], Robert Beshara [2018], Ilan Kapoor, Jamil Khader [2013], and Zahi Zalloua [2019] argue, in different ways, with respect to Žižek). In terms of the colonial underside of Lacan, what is the Algerian context for his discussion of *Antigone* in *Seminar VII* (1959–60), or the Paul Cladual's *Coûfontaine* trilogy in *Seminar VIII* (1960–61), for example? Roudinesco tells us that Lacan smuggled copies of his notes on *Antigone* to his step-daughter, Laurence Bataille, when she was incarcerated, in May 1960, at Prison de la Roquette on charges of raising funds for the FLN, Algerian freedom fighters (187). Is there an anti-colonial connection to be made between the heroine and the step-daughter? Certainly Sophocles' play, which is not to say Lacan's interpretation, has been an important source for anti-colonial drama in African, Palestinian, and Indigenous North American contexts.[3]

And, in *Seminar VIII*, Lacan's description of the Algerian colonial context in Claudel's *Coûfontaine* is clear, if fleeting: a character "has just returned from Algeria – a country that has taken on a certain importance since the time at which the play came out [1911]" (Lacan 2015, 285); what's more, another character "got his education in a place where land was being cleared, but where one did not acquire the land – this is clearly indicated in the text – without rather roughly dispossessing other people" (Lacan 2015, 290). Then, to anticipate the second half of this chapter, in what way does Lacan's "split subject," for instance, extract from Lévi-Strauss' accounts of Northwest Coast (Kwakwākā'wakw) transformer masks? Finally, we need to *not* shy away from drawing on psychoanalytic theory to think in a decolonial way.

This last is because geographies of decolonization entail thinking not merely of an obscene underside or unconscious of the West in terms of colonialism or imperialism, but also that, as Walter Mignolo puts it repeatedly, in *On Decoloniality* and elsewhere, "*coloniality* is a decolonial concept," its purpose "to illuminate the darker side of modernity," and that "coloniality emerges as a constitutive, rather than as a derivative dimension of modernity" (Mignolo and Walsh 2018, 111). That is, we can think of the distortion of thought, what it owes to the non-West, of solidarity and phobias but also a shaking off of dominance, and engaging with the non-West that thinks colonialism versus imperialism, or, to use Indigenous theory, reconciliation versus resurgence, and how all of these are thought of in terms of psychoanalysis (what is a decolonial interpretation of dreams, for instance?). Mignolo's relation to psychoanalysis is fraught: on the one hand, he often compares coloniality by reference to Freud or Lacan's unconscious,[4] but his account of the psychoanalytic cure – which, as he puts it, seeks to "help the analysand to come to terms with the psychological disturbances of modern society and be integrated into it," for example – is in full agreement, perhaps without being aware, with the Lacanian critique of ego psychology (as Fanon well knew). To this chapter's engagement with the Lacan of the 1950s, of the split subject and the L-schema, might be added, were there time, inquiries into the Lacan of the 1960s and 1970s, asking about the role of *jouissance*, the non-relation, the sinthome, of spatial and algebraic theories of knots and mathemes and algorithms (should we re-Arabicize the algorithm, as Ed Finn gestures towards in *What Algorithms Want*, for instance).[5]

But Mignolo, Enrique Dussel, and Beshara can also help us to understand how, in a Lacanian spatial fashion, "decolonization" itself has different registers in different regional struggles. In Canada, the tension between decolonization and its relation to Indigenization has been articulated, not in unproblematic fashion, by Eve Tuck and L. Wayne Yang (2012, 2014), Leanne Betasamosake Simpson (2014), Audra Simpson (2014), and Glenn Coulthard (2014) that are coded as either identity politics or land and sovereignty in a way resistant to a decolonial cosmopolitanism. But in the Global

South, the decolonial, as Mignolo and Dussel argue with respect to "darker sides" and "transmodernity," denotes a shrugging off – but also perhaps an orientation towards the colonial heritage – or what in other very different contexts (Gilroy 2006; Žižek 2000) is called postcolonial melancholy. Then, in the Maghreb and the West, "decolonization" is also a signifier of a critical reading that, following Said's *Orientalism* (1979) and *Cultural and Imperialism* (1993), seeks out non-Western inflections in the Eurocentric canon. Beshara (2018) thus adopts Laura Marks' (2012) contention that in order to decolonize European philosophy, one must "rediscover its Islamic . . . origins," for example, "in order to decolonize psychoanalysis and psychoanalyze Islam" (Beshara 2018, 104–105).

Here we can also trace two trajectories in social and decolonial psychoanalytic thinking: first, Edward Said's argument, in *Freud and the Non-European* (2003), that "Freud was an explorer of the mind, of course, but also, in the philosophical sense, an overturner and a re-mapper of accepted or settled geographies and genealogies" (27). Freud's overturning and re-mapping is not about some sunny optimism, as is made clear in the well-known passage on "the narcissism of minor differences," from *Group Psychology and the Analysis of the Ego* (1921), where he "scales up" from the couple-form to the family and then "when men come together in larger units," and so:

> Of two neighbouring towns each is the other's most jealous rival; every little canton looks down upon the others with contempt. Closely related races keep one another at arm's length; the South German cannot endure the North German, the Englishman casts every kind of aspersion upon the Scot, the Spaniard despises the Portuguese. We are no longer astonished that greater differences should lead to an almost insuperable repugnance, such as the Gallic people feel for the German, the Aryan for the Semite, and the white races for the coloured.
>
> (SE XVIII 101)

This is of course a strong tradition in psychoanalysis – especially the themes of the neighbor and the narcissism of small differences, and Said's melancholy reminder elsewhere that "anti-Semitism" should include Arab-phobia, or debates in Canadian contexts over Indigeneity, the Métis nation, and Kwakwākā'wakw totems on Coast Salish lands remind us that it is not only in Freud's (mostly) European examples that we can find such problematics.[6]

The *geographies* of Lacanian thought, then, connect its production in the metropolitan center, and how it was informed, and taken up, in however distorted a fashion by anti-colonial movements and cultures, but also the spatial dimensions of that thought itself. If we are accustomed to think of the "other" as a negative category of subjectivity, a decolonial psychoanalysis helps us to think of the other in a properly spatial way. And we can see how the "other" as demarcated in decolonial discourses is quite different from the various others of psychoanalysis in Enrique Dussel and Alessandro Fornazzari's 2002 essay "World-System and Trans-Modernity," where "exteriority" is seen as the transmodern or world system "other" to postmodernism qua totality:

> the metacategory "exteriority" can illuminate an analysis of the cultural "positivity" not included by modernity, an analysis based not on postmodernity's suppositions but rather on those of what I have called "trans"-modernity. That is to say, exteriority is a process that takes off, originates, and mobilizes itself from an "other" place . . . than European and North American modernity.
>
> (234)

Evidently what Dussel and Fornazzari are working out here is a dialectical critique of the negative "othering," a critique that returns by demarcating a decolonial exteriority that, as they argue, "takes off, originates, and mobilizes itself from an 'other' place" that is exterior to "European and North American modernity." For the Argentinian-Mexican Dussel, then, the other is both marked by the metropole, by the colonizer, and a space that marks *other than*: the decolonial subject is both othered and othering, a *de*-colonial subject that is spatially different from the postcolonial (in some ways to do with Latin American versus African/South Asian demarcations of postcolonialism); but can, thanks to the work of Tuck and Yang (2012), be connected to current debates in decolonial theory with respect to, on the one hand, "Indigenization" and, on the other, "reconciliation." In a North American context, or what is called Turtle Island, if "always indigenize" has come to seem as impossible an injunction as Freud argued was the biblical demand that we love our neighbor, so too the putatively more radical "decolonize," which, as Tuck and Yang (2012) have argued, is *not a metaphor*. Decolonizing is not simply a matter of changing the curriculum, or hiring more Indigenous scholars, of changing structures and credentializing, nor – and this is germane to our discussion of how Northwest Coast masks end up informing Lacanian theory – thinking about research protocols.[7]

Here I want to make a nod to questions of methodology or historiography, drawing first on David Pavón-Cuéllar and Ian Parker's (2013) argument that Lacanian discourse analysis does not regard material "as analyzable discourses to be analysed by us, but as *analysing discourses*," which is to say that they "do not adopt a position outside the material in order to 'apply' the analysis to it," but instead pay attention to how "the narrative reflects and makes sense of itself" – just as "in Lacanian psychoanalysis, it is the 'analysand' who analyses," they treat their narratives "as reflexive, self-critical discourses that return on themselves and 'analyse' themselves" (315–316).[8] I want to continue this intervention by paying more attention to *the split or barred subject* and tracing its genealogy to specific Indigenous cultural objects. I do so by reading two specific moments in Lacan's *Écrits*, from the 1958/60 talk "Remarks on Daniel Lagache's Presentation" and the 1958 review "The Youth of Gide, or the Letter and Desire." The question I am asking here, then, is in what way does Lacan's "split subject" extract specifically from Claude Lévi-Strauss' accounts of Northwest Coast (Kwakiutl, or what are now called Kwakwākā'wakw) transformer masks and, generally, from his anthropological approach to form? In "Remarks," Lacan describes how a "figure joins together two profiles whose unity is tenable only if the mask remains closed" (2006, 562), and in "Youth," after referring to Freud on the "*Spaltung* or splitting of the ego," he asks "Must I . . . show them how to handle a mask that unmasks the face it represents only by splitting in two" (2006, 633). Footnotes to these passages, from both Lacan (for "Youth") and Bruce Fink (for his translation of "Remarks"), direct the reader to two texts by Lévi-Strauss: his 1943 essay on "The Art of the Northwest Coast," and "Split Representation in the Art of Asia and America," which first appeared in book form in 1958. Reading Lacan with Lévi-Strauss, then, allows us to trace a genealogy of the split subject, from mask to anthropologist to psychoanalyst – but to what end? In what way can or should we read the theory of the split subject – which evidently owes much, on the one hand, to a structuralist theory of the sign, and the *barre* between signifier and signified, and, on the other, to Freud's *Spaltung* and to Lacan's heterodox splitting of the Ideal-Ego and Ego-Ideal, or the *sujet d'énoncé* and *sujet d'enunciation* – as originating in mask making or colonial anthropology? Am I arguing that Lacan has colonized Indigenous artefacts for his European theory? Or does this reading demonstrate how Kwakiutl art works turn out to anticipate a key tenet of structuralism? Or, finally, does my method here – tracing influence via Lacan and Lévi-Strauss' – argue for a textual decolonization of psychoanalysis?

We can see this by turning to colonial (nineteenth-century) and decolonial (contemporary) iterations of the split subject, exploring how the turn to formalization in Lacan is both a spatial algorithm and a conceptual decolonization.[9] That is, formalization, whether the split subject or the matheme, is a matter of an *already-existing* formalization among *les damnées*. We can see this in the historical and contemporary transformer masks by Haida, Tsimshian, Kwakwākā'wakw, and Nuxalk artists. Lévi-Strauss (1982) describes the masks' machinic mechanisms as a "system of ropes, pulleys, and hinges [that] can cause mouths to mock a novice's terrors, eyes to mourn his death, beaks to devour him" (7).[10] And Franz Boas describes how in a Kwakwākā'wakw "representation of a killer whale (*Orca sp.*), the animal has been split along its whole back towards the front," adding that the "two profiles of the head have been joined."[11] Lévi-Strauss also notes in a passage Lacan points us to in a note to "Jeunesse de Gide,"

> They hold at the same time the function of masking and unmasking. But when it comes to unmasking, it is the mask which, by a kind of

> reverse splitting, opens up into two halves, while the actor himself is dissociated in the split representation, which aims, as we saw, at flattening out as well as displaying the mask.
>
> (Lévi-Strauss 1967, 256–257)

Lacan stresses how the artifact "joins together two profiles whose unity is tenable only if the mask remains closed," and "the ambiguity of the process" whereby the fantasy of the unity of the subject is established ("la figure du masque, pour être dimidiée, n'est pas symétrique . . . qu'elle conjoint deux profils dont l'unité ne se soutient que de ce que le masque reste fermé") (Lacan 2006, 562).

The dynamics of the masks, then, are paradoxically unstable, both machine-like in their mechanics, but also a *reverse splitting* that is joined, three dimensions that, to meet a graphic requirement, are flattened. How do these plastic descriptions (masks are also ceremonial) accord with Lacan's theory of the split subject? Lacan paraphrases Lagache on the Ego-Ideal and Ideal-Ego in ways that also hew closely to Freud in the *Spaltung* of the Ego essay, and indeed Fink, in his translator's note, argues that Lacan's word *dimidiée* as split denotes "each side being treated or behaving differently."[12] Lacan's discussion in the Gide essay is more metatheoretical, discussing how psychoanalysts mistake the splitting of the ego for a weakness (a colonial notion *in nuce*) and making more explicit reference to masks as discussed by Lévi-Strauss.

Here we have, appropriately enough, two contradictory ideas. First, the orthodox Freudian notion, developed in his late essay on the *Spaltung* of the ego, of entertaining two contradictory thoughts at the same time (the child "responds to the conflict with two contrary reactions, both of which are valid and effective" – Freud SE XXIII 275), which is then exemplified by the masks that split open, or the split artistic representations, described by Lévi-Strauss. A face that splits to reveal another face: so, two faces. Thus, a model for the split subject, which is to be metastasized by Lacan via not only the unconscious, language, and the signifying *barre*, but also (later) by the barred other. Second, we have that spatial splitting also evident in the geographic unconscious, or the question of how those masks and representations make their way into Lacanian theory. The geographic unconscious is always a repression:[13] as noted earlier, it is due to a colonial disavowal (I know very well that the masks and other ceremonial regalia of Indigenous peoples have immense cultural value, if only because they have been so described by my anthropologists and I can sell them to museums, but nonetheless I will ban their use and production). It is the spatiality of that split, or the scaling down from the global to the matheme, that I argue accounts for a connection via the geographic unconscious, between the decolonial other, or *les damnées*, and Lacan's turn to formalization. What these descriptions, and the objects, convey, then, is not a static model; instead we have to ask, as Said puts it, *how does theory travel*?

I want to argue that a formalization of Lacan's that is quite contemporary to his introduction of the split subject, the so-called L-schema, helps us here, for the L-schema stages that very split in a visual and graphic form. That is, the L-schema demonstrates how the split in the subject, first theorized by the Kwakwākā'wakw, is both dynamic and constitutive. How does this work? It means that one way in which to decolonize Lacan's theory is to see his mathemes, algorithms, and graphs as the intrusion of *les damnées* onto the metropolitan scene. This may seem to be a claim with very little evidence, based on a selective reading of a few paragraphs and footnotes to "Remarks on Daniel Lagache's Presentation" and "The Youth of Gide." (Although Lacan is notorious for introducing ideas once – like *das Ding* in *Seminar VII*, and then never returning to it – a casualty of his improvisatory/free associational ways.) But if we read the split subject, the L-schema, globally (or what in *Seminar XIX* is called the "rift in the real," where the transformer masks can be read as "dismantling the machine for the hole that passes thru you," so that "our *not-all* is discordance" – Lacan 2018, 14), the L-schema maps the political via a spatial discordance, as a way of thinking, say, the Kwakwākā'wakw with Lacan. Here the true leap of faith is not to connect the split subject to Indigenous theory but rather to make the move of an *après-coup*, to move backwards in Lacan's theoretical formation, to see the Kwakwākā'wakw mask as an example of what Robinson called Fanon's radical anticipations. The L-schema is one of Lacan's earliest formalizations, from May 1955, just a month after the Bandung Conference (a key moment in the decolonial struggle),[14] and three years before the Lagache paper (see Figure 3.1).

There are any number of excellent readings of the L-schema, including those of Bruce Fink in his *Clinical Introduction* (1997), Derek Hook (2018), and Darian Leader (2000). Leader situates his genealogy of the L-schema in the development of formalizations in philosophy and mathematics in the mid-twentieth century. Crucially, he convincingly shows that Lacan's L-schema originates in both cybernetics and anthropology, in both Shannon Weaver's 1949 diagram of transmitted and received symbols *and* Lévi-Strauss'

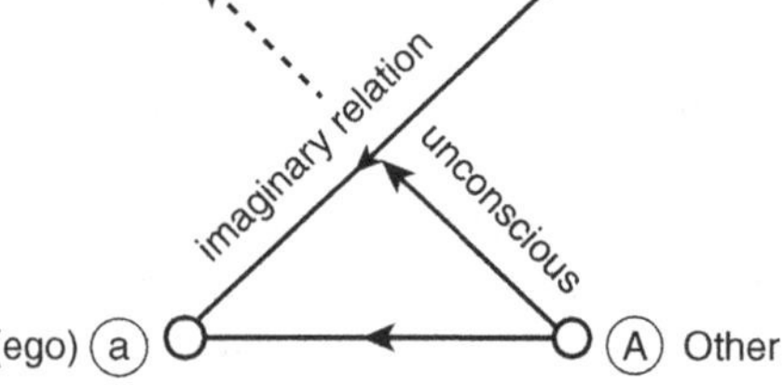

Figure 3.1 L-schema, in Lacan (1991, 243)

model for kinship.[15] Fink, in a comment that recalls Anne Anlin Cheng's argument that "intrasubjectivity exists as a form of intersubjectivity and that intersubjectivity often speaks in the voice of intrasubjectivity" (Cheng 2000, 28), notes that the four places of the L-schema, "ego, alter-ego, subject, and Other," can be found within the individual and also "used to understand the imaginary and symbolic components of the analytic relationship" (Fink 1997, 252 n. 64).

I want to quickly sketch out how to read the L-schema in two different ways: first, its orthodox Lacanian meaning, and second, a decolonial reading. Lacan argues that our subjectivity is constituted by the imaginary versus symbolic/unconscious, but what is key to the schema is that they are not just different axes but that they also cross. In the 1950s, when the role of the clinic is to move the analysand from the imaginary to the symbolic, Lacan is still positing a constitutive antagonism. That is, the imaginary is the noise effecting the message of the big Other. And if the L-schema is, in Lacanian terms, essentially about the Lacan of the imaginary, of recognition, and is not properly speaking the Lacan of the signifier, of the symbolic, let alone the real, then we cannot neglect the shame that Lacanians have when they return to early Lacan, to the mirror stage (we sneer at our colleagues who only ever teach the mirror stage essay) – a shame that is, properly speaking, every bit as colonial as those Lévi-Strauss castigated for their "archaic illusions" – theories of the mirror stage and the imaginary are a "primitivism" for Lacanians. I propose that we move beyond respecting such a stage-ism of Lacan, precisely in favor of a narrativization of his work, which simultaneously proposes a historicist approach (the 1950s are the imaginary, and so on – J-A. Miller, Žižek) *and* a Whiggish theory of Lacan (he gets more difficult, the real Lacan is that of the 1970s, the *semblant*, knots, Sade-like dissolution – Edelman). Such a move would resist the tendency in Lacanian theory towards university discourse and, too, respect the reality that *we do not read Lacan in chronological order* – such a historical narrative is always constituted *après-coup*, after the fact, in the same way that the L-schema, invented contemporaneously with the Bandung Conference, contains the germs of earlier Kwakwākā'wakw masks *before* they make their citational appearance in the Lagache and Gide essays.[16]

The L-schema proposes *two splits* – the split between the speaking subject (S) and the ego, and the split between the ego and the little other: these we can return to the global split, to the geographic unconscious, that "rift in the real" or the axes of imaginary and symbolic as what Dolar (2009) notes is "variously named as conflictuality, antagonism, rift, a crack in the social tissue, an excess, the point of ambivalence, untying of social bonds, negativity" in the mask, in the formalization, in the global real. This second split, this second spatiality, one of the global, I propose we call a matter of discordance (to cite an important term in the later Lacan [2018] – in *Seminar XIX*), after an artwork spelling out the word "DISCORDANCY," by the

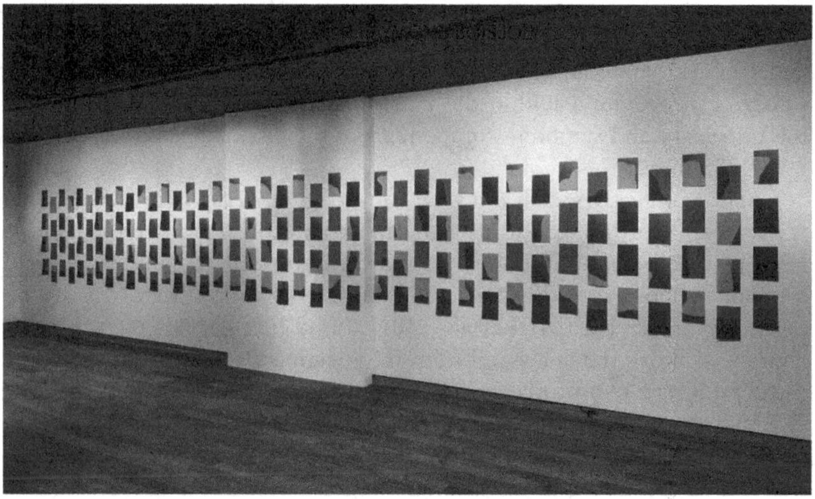

Figure 3.2 Raymond Boisjoly, *newer figures of another fleeting (non) relation* (photocopies, staples, dimensions variable, 2017)

Indigenous (Québecois-Haida) artist Raymond Boisjoly, to see how well Lacan's algorithm or formalization maps the political via a spatial discordance. Boisjoly's artwork (Figure 3.2) is titled *newer figures of another fleeting (non) relation* (2017) and renders the sign or letter of the signifier "DISCORDANCY") into an image that refuses meaning, refuses to coalesce, marking on the space of the gallery wall (rendering the institutional space into the picture plane of the aesthetic).

The 160 fragments of the Lacanian letter (spelling out "DISCORDANCY") that make up Boisjoly's work also posit a spatiality, an illusion of three dimensions, that does two things. One, Boisjoly's spatiality reaches back to and reverses the flattening of three dimensions that Boas and Lévi-Strauss find constitutive of the split representations; two, that spatiality also anticipates the turn from two dimensions to three in the later Lacan's topologies. This spatiality also inscribes the geographic decolonial, and so with the help of Boisjoly's non-relation/discordancy, we can decolonize the L-schema (Figure 3.3).

Now the ego = colonizer, caught up in an imaginary relation with the colonized: this is the politics of recognition, of the spectacle. Decoloniality, then, is the big Other, the insistence on a politics of revolt and resurgence, which interpellates the split subject qua discordancy. This is hardly a triumphalist reading, however, as Boisjoly's notes on the artworks' material ("photocopies, staples, dimensions variable") suggest – no heroic masterpiece here; this is not canvas and oil or marble, but is made of far humbler

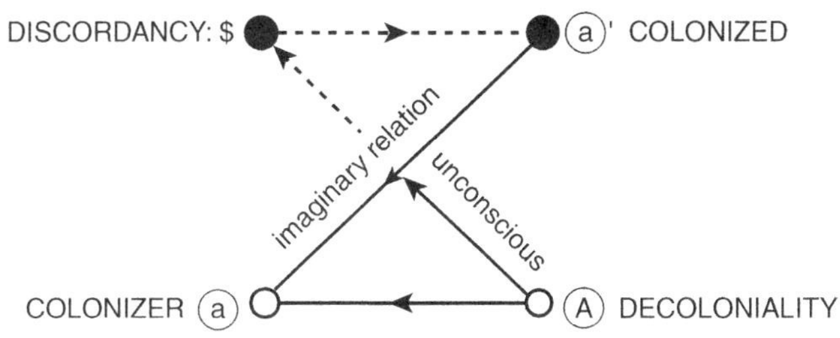

Figure 3.3 Decolonial L-schema

stuff. And, as Derek Hook (2018) reminds us in his comments on the original L-schema, this is to be expected "given the psychoanalytic emphasis on the split nature of the subject and upon the fleeting quality of unconscious events which suddenly emerge and then disappear" (35). Determining that Lacan's split subject has Indigenous origins will not satisfy radicals who see psychoanalysis as merely therapy, but it may help us to understand why that which we do not anticipate is more welcome than that which we do.

Notes

1 Lewis Gordon (1995) also discusses Fanon and Robinson on Fanon in his chapter "Fanon's Continued Relevance" (85–103).

2 To this survey of Fanon criticism should also be added the recent work of David Marriott (2018, 2021) and Gautam Basu Thakur (2021).

3 See, for one discussion, James Gibb's article "*Antigone* and her African Sisters: West African Versions of a Greek Original" in Gillespie (2007).

4 Mignolo often juxtaposes Freud's unconscious alongside Marx's surplus value: *On Decoloniality* 10, 140, 142, 252.

5 "An algorithm is a recipe, an instruction set, a sequence of tasks to achieve a particular calculation or result, like the steps required to calculate a square root or tabulate the Fibonacci sequence. The word itself derives from Abū 'Abdallāh Muhammad ibn Mūsā al-Khwārizmī, the famed ninth-century CE mathematician (from whose name algebra is also derived). *Algorismus* was originally the process for calculating Hindu-Arabic numerals. Via al-Kwārizmī, the algorithm was associate with the revolutionary concepts of positional notation, the decimal point, and zero." Ed Finn, 2017 (kindle loc. 358). Beshara (2019) engages with the later Lacan, citing Lacan on how repetition engenders *jouissance*, how "the endless repetition of the master signifier . . . produces the interpellated ($) who has no choice but to keep endlessly *desiring* for freedom (*a*), while indulging in *jouissance* (JΦ)" (54).

6 Said in *Orientalism*: "'Semites' were not only the Jews but the Muslims as well" (Said, 1979, 99) and his more poetic, "by an almost inescapable logic, I have found myself writing the history of a strange, secret sharer of Western anti-Semitism" (Said, 1979, 27). See also Beshara (2021). For discussions of *métissage* in Canadian contexts, see Chris Anderson's *Métis: Race, Recognition, and the Struggle for Indigenous Peoplehood* (2014) and Jordan Abel's *Nishga* (2021). In Vancouver, historian Jean Barman (2007)

writes that the "erasure of Indigeneity" from the city in the early twentieth century was accompanied by a compromise formation, as it were: "the replacement of indigenous Indigeneity with a sanitized Indigeneity from elsewhere," so Kwakwākā'wakw totem poles replace the Squamish settlements of X̱wáy̓x̱way (26).

7 Indeed, I was making remarks along these lines at a Critical Psychology Congress (Northern New Mexico College, 2019) when I was reminded of Audre Lorde's imperative that "the master's tools will never dismantle the master's house," to which I answered that I thought of the "master" in that context not as European theorists but rather the forces of capital. Of course, for some interlocutors, this will not satisfy, since in Lorde's original context (a 1979 intervention at the NYU Institute for the Humanities *Second Sex* Conference) she was critiquing white feminists for their lack of knowledge of poor, lesbian, women of color; furthermore, Lacan easily fits into what have variously been called *les maitres de penseur* or even Ricouer's "masters of suspicion." (Note that Lorde was remarking on the need for Black voices in a conference on de Beauvoir; further, she also makes the following very Lacan-friendly comment: "what about interracial cooperation between feminists who don't love each other?") And, too, I would argue that Lacanian theory holds much for the emancipatory project, for the decolonizing project, *precisely* because of his theories of the *master* signifier and their role in our unconscious, as well as his four discourses, including the *master's* discourse. Beshara notes that he "works with the question of the master not as a person but as a signifier, and this is the psychoanalytic question, of course, because regardless of where we come from certain master signifiers are dominant in our unconscious, which forms our subjectivity in certain ways" (personal communication).

8 While this notion of discourses analyzing themselves is not without controversy, I suggest that it is similar to Marxist, and especially Adorno's, notions of immanent critique. Derek Hook has remarked (in a personal communication): "Frankly, while I like the idea on paper, it doesn't really seem feasible to me. Sure, an analysand can, in the context of the clinic, offer analyzing comments on their own speech and process, but this doesn't really seem viable in the context of written discourse."

9 It is worth reminding the reader unfamiliar with the colonial history (and present) of Canada that from 1885 to 1951, the Canadian government forbade Indigenous people from performing sacred rituals, including the potlatch. The irony is that it was precisely the potlatch that would, via Marcel Mauss' description in *Le Don,* come to so fascinate French intellectuals (including André Breton, the Situationists, who named their 1950s newsletter *Potlatch*, and Bataille). Masks and other ceremonial regalia were seized by the federal government and then sold to museums around the world; and so because of these colonial strictures the masks came to be in New York museums, and hence seen by Claude Lévi-Strauss. For a novelization of these proceedings by an Indigenous writer, see Clutesi (1969). Knight (2018) argues that Clutesi's novel is a literary refusal to reveal. See also Bracken (1997).

10 *The Way of the Masks,* citing his "The Art of the Northwest Coast at the Museum of Natural History," *Gazette des Beaux-Arts,* 1943, 175–182.

11 Franz Boas, *Primitive Art*. Instituttet for *Sammenlignende Kulturforskning*, series B, Vol III (Oslo: 1927), 239, in Lévi-Strauss (1967, 248).

12 I also hear "mi-dis" or what is half-said at mid-day – the later Lacan of *Encore* (1998), as in the truth "of the half-telling [*mi-dire*]" (93).

13 I discuss the concept of the "geographic unconscious" in my chapter "Always Geographize! Fredric Jameson and Political Space." In Friederike Landau et al. (eds.), *(Un)Grounding: Post-Foundational Interventions in Space*. Frankfurt: transcript 2021.

14 Richard Wright's *The Color Curtain* (1956), a journalistic account of the Bandung Conference, is notable not only for its range of reference, from the legacy of 350 years of Dutch colonialism in Indonesia, where the conference was held, to the sense of foreboding with which Western media viewed this unprecedented gathering of newly decolonized Asian and African countries, and such gems as a list of Malay phrases for Dutch overseers: "Sweep up the front first," "All my stolen property has been returned," "You are stupid" (Wright, 1956, 180–181). Wright also recounts explaining to a white American woman why her Black roommate was using skin-lightening chemicals, in terms reminiscent of Fanon: "Negroes have been made ashamed of being black. Dark Hindus feel the same way. White people have made them feel like that. The American Negroes are black and they live in a white country. Almost every picture and image they see is white. . . . Every day that woman commits psychological suicide" (186–187).

15 All three diagrams, shown in Leader (177–178), are squares, crossing in the middle. Markos Zafiropoulos, in his volume on Lacan and Lévi-Strauss (2010), makes the connection even stronger, citing Lacan's 2 May 1956 address to the *Société française de Philosophie* in which he discussed trying to "apply this grid to the symptom in obsessional neurosis" (Zafiropoulos 168: see also 170, where Zafiropoulos shows a Lévi-Strauss grid side by side with the L-schema).

16 Just as Lacan (2006) draws on the seven years (1788–1795) between Kant's *Critique of Practical Reason* and Sade's *Philosophy in the Boudoir*, to argue the latter "yields the truth of the Critique" (646), so we can note that the contemporaneity of Bandung and the L-schema *anticipates* the arrival of the Kwakwākā'wakw masks, via the potlatch ban, Boas, and Lévi-Strauss. One reviewer of an earlier draft of this chapter suggested that the point of the L-schema is precisely to provide a map of communicative interaction, and a guide to how the imaginary intersubjectivity of everyday conversation should be avoided in the clinical domain where precisely the axis of Other-*Es* is to be prioritized. But this a priori would miss the argument, in this paragraph, for a constitutive antagonism and, indeed, an argument for the dialectics of the imaginary as the noise effecting the message of the big Other.

Works Cited

Abel, Jordon. 2021. *Nishga.* Toronto: McClelland and Stewart.

Almond, Ian. 2012. "Anti-Capitalist Objections to the Postcolonial: Some Conciliatory Remarks on Žižek and Context." *Ariel: A Review of International English Literature* 43.1: 1–21.

Anderson, Chris. 2014. *Métis: Race, Recognition, and the Struggle for Indigenous Peoplehood.* Vancouver: UBC Press.

Barman, Jean. 2007. "Erasing Indigenous Indigeneity in Vancouver." *B.C. Studies* 155 (Autumn): 3–30.

Basu Thakur, Gautam. 2021. "Fanon's 'Zone of Non-Being': Blackness and the Politics of the Real." Sheldon George and Derek Hook, eds., *Lacan and Race: Racism, Identity and Psychoanalytic Theory.* London: Routledge.

Beshara, Robert. 2018. "Decolonizing Psychoanalysis/Psychoanalyzing Islamophobia." Ian Parker and Sabah Siddiqui, eds. *Islamic Psychoanalysis and Psychoanalytic Islam: Cultural and Clinical Dialogues.* London: Routledge, 102–117.

———. 2019. *Decolonial Psychoanalysis: Towards Critical Islamophobia Studies.* New York: Routledge.

———. 2021. *Freud and Said: Contrapuntal Psychoanalysis as Liberation Praxis*. London: Palgrave.

Bhabha, Homi. 1986. "Remembering Fanon: Self, Psyche and the Colonial Condition." In Fanon 1986, xxi–xxxvii.

———. 1996. "Day by Day . . . with Frantz Fanon." In Read 1996, 186–205.

Bjelić, Dušan I. 2016. "Freud's Conquest and the Balkans' Orientalist Phantasmagoria." *Intoxication, Modernity, and Colonialism*. New York: Palgrave Macmillan, 189–245.

Bracken, Christopher. 1997. *The Potlatch Papers: A Colonial Case History*. Chicago: University of Chicago Press.

Cheng, Anne Anlin. 2000. *The Melancholy of Race: Psychoanalysis, Assimilation, and Hidden Grief*. New York: Oxford University Press.

Clarke, Simon. 2003. "Colonial Identity and Ethnic Hatred: Fanon, Lacan and Zizek." *Social Theory, Psychoanalysis and Racism*. London: Macmillan, 99–122.

Clutesi, George. 1969. *Potlatch*. Sydney: Gray.

Coulthard, Glen Sean. 2014. *Red Skin White Masks: Rejecting the Colonial Politics of Recognition*. Minneapolis: University of Minnesota Press.

Dabashi, Hamid. 2013. "Can Non-Europeans Think?" *al-jazeera.com*, 15 January. Accessed 27 October 2019.

———. 2016. *Can Non-Europeans Think?* London: Zed.

Derrida, Jacques. 1998. "Geopsychoanalysis: ' . . . and the Rest of the World'." Christopher Lane, ed. *Psychoanalysis and Race*. New York: Columbia University Press, 65–90.

Dolar, Mladen. 2009. "Freud and the Political." *Theory & Event* 12.3.

Dussel, Enrique D. and Alessandro Fornazzari. 2002. "World-System and 'Trans'-Modernity." *Nepantla: Views from South* 3.2: 221–244.

Fanon, Frantz. 1986. *Black Skin, White Masks*. London: Pluto.

Ferreira da Silva, Denise. 2007. *Toward a Global Idea of Race*. Minneapolis: University of Minnesota Press.

Fink, Bruce. 1997. *A Clinical Introduction to Lacanian Psychoanalysis: Theory and Technique*. Cambridge: Harvard University Press.

Finn, Ed. 2017. *What Algorithms Want: Imagination in the Age of Computing*. Cambridge: MIT Press.

Freud, Sigmund. 1921. "Group Psychology and the Analysis of the Ego." *SE* XVIII: 67–143.

Gates, Henry Louis. 1991. "Critical Fanonism." *Critical Inquiry* 17.3: 457–470.

Gillespie, Carol, ed. 2007. *Classics in Post-Colonial Worlds*. Oxford: Oxford University Press.

Gilroy, Paul. 2006. *Postcolonial Melancholia*. New York: Columbia University Press.

Gordon, Lewis R. 1995. *Fanon and the Crisis of European Man: An Essay on Philosophy and the Human Sciences*. London: Routledge.

Hall, Stuart. 1996. "The After-Life of Frantz Fanon: Why Fanon? Why Now? Why *Black Skin, White Mask?*" In Read 1996, 12–37.

Hook, Derek. 2018. *Six Moments in Lacan: Communication and Identification in Psychology and Psychoanalysis*. London: Routledge.

Kapoor, Ilan. 2018. "The Pervert Versus the Hysteric: Politics at Tahrir Square." Ilan Kapoor, ed. *Psychoanalysis and the Global*. Lincoln: University of Nebraska Press, kindle.

Khader, Jamil. 2013. "Žižek's Infidelity: Lenin, the National Question, and the Post-colonial Legacy of Revolutionary Internationalism." Jamil Khader and Molly Anne Rothenberg, eds. *Žižek Now: Current Perspectives in Žižek Studies*. Cambridge: Polity Press, 159–174.

Khanna, Ranjana. 2003. *Dark Continents: Psychoanalysis and Colonialism*. Durham: Duke University Press.

Knight, Natalie. 2018. *Dispossessed Indigeneity: Literary Excavations of Internalized Colonialism*. Ph.D. diss. Vancouver: Simon Fraser University.

Lacan, Jacques. 1981. *The Four Fundamental Concepts of Psychoanalysis. The Seminar of Jacques Lacan, Book XI*. Trans. Alan Sheridan. New York: Norton.

———. 1991. *The Ego in Freud's Theory and in the Technique of Psychoanalysis. The Seminar of Jacques Lacan, Book II*. Trans. Sylvana Tomaselli. New York: Norton.

———. 1998. *Encore: On Feminine Sexuality, the Limits of Love and Knowledge. The Seminar of Jacques Lacan, Book XX*. Trans. Bruce Fink. New York: Norton.

———. 2006. *Écrits*. Trans. Bruce Fink. New York: Norton.

———. 2015. *Transference. The Seminar of Jacques Lacan, Book VII*. Trans. Bruce Fink. Cambridge: Polity Press.

———. 2018. *. . . or Worse. The Seminar of Jacques Lacan, Book XIX*. Trans. A.R. Price. Cambridge: Polity Press.

Leader, Darian. 2000. "The Schema L." Bernard Burgoyne, ed. *Drawing the Soul: Schemas and Diagrams in Psychoanalysis*. London: Routledge, 172–189.

Lévi-Strauss, Claude. 1967. "Split Representation in the Art of Asia and America." *Structural Anthropology*. Trans. Claire Jacobson and Brooke Grundfest Schoepf. New York: Anchor, 239–263.

———. 1982. *The Way of the Masks*. Trans. Sylvia Modelski. Seattle: University of Washington Press.

Lorde, Audre. 1984. "The Master's Tools Will Never Dismantle the Master's House." *Sister Outsider: Essays and Speeches*. Berkeley: Crossing Press, 110–114.

Marks, Laura. 2012. "A Deleuzian Ijtihad: Unfolding Deleuze's Islamic Sources Occulted in the Ethnic Cleansing of Spain." A. Salanha and J.M. Adams, eds. *Deleuze and Race*. Edinburgh: Edinburgh University Press, 51–72.

Marriott, D.S. 2018. *Whither Fanon? Studies in the Blackness of Being*. Binghamton: SUNY Press.

———. 2021. *Lacan Noir: Lacan and Afro-Pessimism*. London: Palgrave.

Mignolo, Walter. 2013. "Yes, We Can: Non-European Thinkers and Philosophers." *aljazeera.com*, 19 February. Accessed 27 October 2019.

Mignolo, Walter and Catherine E. Walsh, eds. 2018. *On Decoloniality: Concepts, Analytics, Praxis*. Durham: Duke University Press.

Parry, Benita. 1987. "Problems in Current Theories of Colonial Discourse." *Oxford Literary Review* 9.1–2: 27–58.

Pavón-Cuéllar, David and Ian Parker. 2013. "From the White Interior to an Exterior Blackness: A Lacanian Discourse Analysis of Apartheid Narratives." Garth Stevens et al., eds. *Race, Memory and the Apartheid Archive: Towards a Transformative Psychosocial Praxis*. London: Palgrave, 315–332.

Read, Alan. 1996. *The Fate of Blackness: Frantz Fanon and Visual Representation*. London/Seattle: ICA/Bay Press.

Robinson, Cedric. 1993. "The Appropriation of Frantz Fanon." *Race and Class* 35.1: 79–91.

———. 2000. *Black Marxism: The Making of the Black Radical Tradition*. Chapel Hill: University of North Carolina Press.

Rose, Jacqueline. 1996. *States of Fantasy*. New York: Oxford University Press.

Roudinesco, Elisabeth. 1997. *Jacques Lacan*. Trans. Barbara Bray. New York: Columbia University Press.

Said, Edward. 1979. *Orientalism*. New York: Vintage.

———. 1993. *Culture and Imperialism*. New York: Vintage.

———. 2003. *Freud and the Non-European*. London: Verso.

Sanborn, A. 2009. "The Reunification of the Kwakwaka'wakw Mask with Its Cultural Soul." *Museum International* 61: 81–86.

Seshadri-Crooks, Kalpana. 2000. *Desiring Whiteness: A Lacanian Analysis of Race*. New York: Routledge.

Simpson, Audra. 2014. *Mohawk Interruptus: Political Life Across the Borders of Settler States*. Durham: Duke University Press.

Simpson, Leanne Betasamosake. 2014. "Land as Pedagogy: Nishnaabeg Intelligence and Rebellious Transformation." *Decolonization: Indigeneity, Education & Society* 3.3: 1–25.

Terada, Rei. 2019. "Hegel's Racism for Radicals." *Radical Philosophy* 2.05 (Fall): 11–22.

Tuck, Eve and K. Wayne Yang. 2012. "Decolonization Is Not a Metaphor." *Decolonization: Indigeneity, Education & Society* 1.1: 1–40.

———. 2014. "R-words: Refusing Research." D. Paris and M.T. Winn, eds. *Humanizing Research: Decolonizing Qualitative Inquiry with Youth and Communities*. Thousand Oaks, CA: SAGE, 223–248.

Wright, Richard. 1956. *The Color Curtain: A Report on the Bandung Conference*. Cleveland: World.

Zabala, Santiago. 2012. "Slavoj Žižek and the Role of the Philosopher." *al-jazeera.com*, 25 December. Accessed 27 October 2019.

Zafiropolous, Markos. 2010. *Lacan and Lévi-Strauss or The Return to Freud (1951–1957)*. Trans. John Holland. London: Karnac.

Zallouha, Zahi. 2019. "Decolonial Particularity or Abstract Universalism? No, Thanks! The Case of the Palestinian Question." *The International Journal of Žižek Studies* 13.1: 83–120.

Žižek, Slavoj. 2000. "Melancholy and the Act." *Critical Inquiry* 26.4: 657–681.

———. 2016. "A Reply to My Critics." *The Philosophical Salon*, 5 August. Accessed 27 October 2019.

Chapter 4

Dwelling on the Direction of the Treatment for the Homeless Subject[1]

Chris Vanderwees

Introduction

In Canada and the United States, contemporary psychoanalysis has the reputation of being accessible only for society's educated or elite class, at an immense financial cost where the privatized treatment is likely to last for many years (at two to five appointments per week). This caricature conveys the widespread perception of psychoanalysis in the social imaginary as a discipline detached from the progressive ideals of social responsibility, institutional psychotherapy, and community mental health. In contrast to this misperception, Freud and his early followers, including Alfred Adler, August Aichorn, Siegfried Bernfeld, Erik Erikson, Anna Freud, Eduard Hitschmann, Willi Hoffer, and Wilhelm Reich, helped to establish outpatient clinics for people who could not otherwise afford treatment in ten cities and seven countries across Europe, including Berlin, Budapest, Frankfurt, London, and Vienna, between the world wars from 1918 to 1938. Elizabeth Ann Danto has documented the efforts of these practitioners in *Freud's Free Clinics*.[2] Despite the significance of this psychoanalytic social justice effort of the past, there is little written from the perspective of any psychoanalytic orientation about work with people who are simultaneously marginalized, impoverished, addicted, and homeless.[3]

In this chapter, I would like to dwell on the direction of treatment for those who are without dwelling. Perhaps I can only arrive at a few thoughts about this direction indirectly. I will try to tell you something about the context of my clinical work within a community of the poor and homeless, because I do not think psychoanalysis can be done from an outside office in these circumstances. The analyst cannot always remain on the "sidelines" (as Lacan says), and I believe this work must happen from within the community. Before going further, however, let me first acknowledge this suffix, "less," since the signifier of the "homeless" explicitly indicates a loss. The suffix precisely designates the state or quality of not having or being free from the very thing denoted by the preceding element. This "less" may involve a brutal subtraction that leaves a person destitute but may also

DOI: 10.4324/9781003212072-5

indicate liberation from unbearable circumstances – a loss in either case. I am not talking about metaphors. When I write of the homeless subject, I refer to actual people who live outdoors exposed to Canadian winters, who sleep in tents and shelters, who are in halfway homes, who are shuffled around in foster placements, who seek asylum or arrive on refugee status having fled war, who perpetually couch-surf and ride waves of uncertainty, who escape domestic violence, or who may feel for any myriad of reasons that the place of home collapsed due to devastating family circumstances. I will also say that not all of my analysands at the mission are presently unhoused, but most have experienced prolonged periods of homelessness at some point in their lives. Many live in the squalor of community housing, where the highly overdetermined signifier of the home does not necessarily have a "sweet home" signified. Homelessness is an experience of "displacement" in both the psychoanalytic and phenomenological senses of the word. There really is no place like home, but especially when home is no place.

In the reflections that follow, I am oriented by a few questions in light of work with analysands who are unable to abide an abode due to multiple and interconnected contingencies of poverty, trauma, and addiction that form each singular circumstance of destitution or brokenness. How can psychoanalysis listen to the discourse of the homeless subject? How might we hear the Thing that is *unheimlich* or unhomely in homelessness? And how might one begin to think about the direction of the treatment when working within a community of poverty where many of the analysands are living in circumstances of precarious housing? I begin with a brief commentary on psychoanalytic research on poverty, followed by several reflections on my observations as a practicing psychoanalyst and psychotherapist within St. John the Compassionate, a Christian Orthodox mission and therapeutic community on the lower eastside of Toronto, Canada. I highlight the importance of therapeutic labor and open-ended psychoanalytic treatment in this organization while trying to express how an analyst should not defensively withdraw one's desire to listen in the face of people who are homeless and impoverished (which would only reveal the resistance of the analyst) but can instead deploy an ethics given some variations to the more "classical" psychoanalytical frame so that the homeless subject is able to speak about one's own suffering.

Psychoanalytic Literature on Poverty (or the Resistance of the Analyst)

Emerging from the anti-psychiatry movement in France in the 1950s, institutional psychotherapy, which is also influenced by the work of Lacan and Foucault as well as the Marxist tradition, has significant potential for rethinking work with homeless and impoverished populations.[4] As a psychiatric reform movement, institutional psychotherapy proposes a radical reorganization of the mental health clinic whereby patients actively participate in the management of the facility and its operations, reversing hierarchical structures and shifting power dynamics. This movement's approach, however, is most often associated with clinics for psychosis and is less commonly extended to thinking about the clinical implications of treatment with people experiencing homelessness and poverty who may be suffering from a variety of mental health diagnoses (Mackie 154–155).[5] Further, Lacan's thinking and French psychoanalysis have not historically permeated American and British psychiatric and psychoanalytic institutions.

In a survey of over 70 years of psychoanalytic research, Manasi Kumar explores the discourse of historical psychoanalytic literature on poverty and the poor, accessible through the American Psychoanalytic Electronic Publishing Archive (PEP Web Archive), which consists of a database aggregation of dozens of journals affiliated with the International Psychoanalytic Association and various academic institutions around the world in English, French, German, Greek, Italian, Romanian, Spanish, and Turkish. Kumar does not mention the French institutional psychotherapy movement. She also does not mention the British schools of anti-psychiatry associated with R. D. Laing and David Cooper, which influenced the notion of the therapeutic community. Such a community usually advances group treatment from a perspective of social collectivism and democratic organization where patients (usually referred to as "residents" in the therapeutic community model) are involved in the decision-making processes and day-to-day operations of the clinical organization. Therapeutic communities have been historically implemented for cases of long-term mental health issues, personality disorders, and addictions, but contemporary research from a psychoanalytic perspective in this area is also significantly lacking since the early work of psychiatrists Robert Hirshelwood and Nick Manning.[6] From her assessment of major psychoanalytic journals in the PEP Web Archive, Kumar writes that "most of the writings on poverty come from the American ego psychology school or its hybrid versions such as intersubjectivist, self psychological, and developmental branches of psychoanalysis" (18).

Kumar's rhetorical assessment of analytic literature throughout the PEP Web Archive is that this literature frequently conveys an elitist attitude, one that rationalizes the analyst's distance from poverty and resorts to individualistic and fatalistic understandings of intersectional aspects of impoverishment and social adversity. In many studies, Kumar discovers

> an implicit argument that the poor may not have enough intellectual (financial of course!) and emotional resources to approach and if they did so to sustain deep analytic work. There were suggestions that psychoanalysis may not be the best remedy for people such as the poor who need immediate relief and contributions that well enhance basic minimum in life much before introducing any psychotherapeutic assistance.

> There are also allusions in the literature to poor prognosis and lower satisfaction of the therapist with the content and quality of analysis.
> (16)

The presumption that a poor or homeless person may not have the intellectual capacity to sustain an analysis does not account for the fact that it takes a great deal of intelligence, "street smarts," to survive life on the street. Assuming that those who are impoverished require basic needs to be met before psychotherapeutic assistance already forecloses the possibility of considering that being able to speak about one's own suffering might also constitute a basic need.

Further, Kumar finds that when psychoanalytic literature does invoke the subject of poverty, it is often through metaphorical language applied to patients. Using poverty as a metaphor to speak about a plethora of conditions, clinicians have shed light on little except their own prejudice in relation to the experience of poverty and homelessness, designating what is Other in the patient through such constructions as, for instance, "psychological poverty," "poverty of imagination," "poverty of symbolic capacity," "poverty of relationships," "poverty of interest," "poverty of emotions," "poverty of sexual function," "poverty of ego," "poverty of dreams," and "religious/moral poverty" (Kumar 6–12). What do we make of the clinician's own phantasies of poverty as displaced into the discourse of symptomatology? It is clear that this emphasis on poverty as metaphor for what is lacking in psychical conditions not only posits a deviation from a problematic construction of normalcy (poor as abnormal or deficient), but also contributes to stigmatization of the poor while confusing actual systemic conditions of poverty with clinical judgments about diagnosis.[7] The metaphorization of the poor as a rhetorical move in clinical writing contributes to the exclusion of those who are marginalized from being so-called good candidates for psychoanalysis. Poverty becomes aligned with what is "unanalyzable." Here, I might suggest that the notion of that which is "unanalyzable" can only be properly defined as a condition or circumstance that results in the clinician's own inability to have patience with patients through listening, especially if, as Allan Frosch writes,

> the analyst's idea about psychoanalysis is an essential variable that contributes to our concept of analyzability. Furthermore, the analyst's ideas are always shaped by desire. Wishes and defenses organize our perception of the world, including the world of who is or is not analyzable.
> (2006, 841)

Does the clinician project and defend against something in his or her pathologization of poverty? Could it be that analysts may not feel at home when listening to the homeless? Suffice to say, there is an enormous gap in psychoanalytic research surrounding clinical treatment of the homeless and the poor. If "there is no other resistance to analysis than that of the analyst himself," as Lacan says, then I cannot help but wonder if psychoanalysts might be rather sheltered when it comes to the subject of homelessness (1958/2006, 497).

Confronted with a shortage of literature on actual poverty and homelessness in the field of analysis, I am reminded of Patricia Gherovici's metaphorical reversal: "One might talk about the psychoanalysis of poverty," but one could perhaps more easily "talk about the poverty of psychoanalysis" ("Psychoanalysis" 221). Like Kumar, Gherovici underscores the apparent exclusion of the poor's access to psychoanalysis and the prejudice involved in the psychoanalytic exclusion of the poor. This especially concerns me since most contemporary social service agencies who work with the poor and homeless only administer pharmaceuticals and the work of "adaptation" and "adjustment" through behavioral treatments that introduce an imposition of compliance and dash the opportunity for the analysand to hear something of his or her own desire in speech. Such agencies are quite effective at extinguishing the patient's own agency. Lacan calls out such notions of guiding the analysand to become more "well-adapted" in the paper that I have in mind at the time of writing, "The Direction of the Treatment and the Principles of Its Power" from 1958. "Well-adapted to what," Lacan writes, "if not to the Other's demand?" (1958/2006, 533).

St. John the Compassionate as Therapeutic Community

For the past several of years, I have held psychoanalytic consultations within St. John the Compassionate, an Orthodox Christian mission situated on the lower eastside of downtown Toronto. Since its opening in 1987, the spiritual Fathers and clergy of this particular mission, some of whom are also registered social workers, have created a welcoming space that provides basic necessities in terms of food, shelter, and clothing and the possibility of a social link throughout the day for those who are living in precarious circumstances. For me, the poverty of the mission is close to home. What I mean is that I am literally a neighbor insofar as I live across the street from the organization. Cracked pavement and streetcar tracks mark a separation between where I live and this work. I am a neighbor but also something of an outlander since I am not a member of the clergy or the parish, though I do serve on staff as a psychoanalyst working alongside the members of the community. We work together. I have an office on the third floor. I have two chairs and a couch. On a busy day, the mission may serve several hundred meals to those who pass through the doors. It is important for the clergy and staff to eat together with the community since, as the rule of the mission highlights, "to set a table is not the same as sharing a meal," and "serving the meals includes the presence of each of us at a table" (St. John 67). Some folks come for pastoral counsel, prayer, and liturgy, but many also come to eat, talk, laugh, cry, sing, or sit together at a table with tea or coffee. People arrive regularly in the midst of a breakdown where others do their best to help with the crisis. It is not always clear if I will see the same people from one day to the next due to the vulnerability, destructiveness, and proximity to death in which some become enwrapped. There is a pile of naloxone kits in my office. There are funerals in the chapel where no immediate family is present. Often a photograph of a familiar person will appear posted to the community bulletin board or on top of the piano in a frame. These are the photographs of the dead. These same photographs are finally rehung on the walls of the main floor office. Sometimes I hold impromptu appointments in this office during the meal programs, surrounded with memento mori. "Who . . . so firmly rooted in the everydayness of human suffering," writes Lacan, "has questioned life as to its meaning – not to say that it has none . . . but to say that it has only one, that in which desire is borne by death?" (*Ecrits* 536). Members of the clergy and staff speak frequently about the transient nature of the community due to the perils of street life. The disorganization of this organization, however, emerges as a crucial element to its functionality. Such disorganization allows for a place, a location, where people may arrive from varied backgrounds, all talks and walks of life, but where everyone shares imaginary and symbolic identifications around an indeterminate notion of community and takes on responsibility for the others within this community. For many who frequent the organization, it is a rare place of safety and refuge.

In the early morning, people sleep on mats on the floor. When they wake up, sometimes we will talk about their dreams over breakfast. Once I asked a man who was overwhelmed with his dreams if he ever wrote them down on paper. "No," he replied, "but I draw them." I found him a piece of paper and a pencil and with an artist's hand he sketched with a fervor the terrifying places and faces that haunt him in his sleep. When he had completed the drawings, I asked him if he felt better. "No," he said, "but the noise in my head stopped."

Labor as Therapeutic

In *To Give a Beautiful Witness: The Rule of St. John the Compassionate*, a text that conveys something of the law of the Father and of the ideals that the organization revolves around, there is reference to the significance of the mustard seed, the practice of paying attention to "some little unexpected miracle . . . discovered in a forgotten corner of our day, a touch of colour in a gray day" (St. John the Compassionate 9). Sometimes we can see the seeds, but analytically we must also attune to what can be heard in the mustard that people bring with them to the mission. This obviously requires listening carefully. Here, a particular branch of Christian ethics intersects with the ideals of institutional psychotherapy, as many of the people who seek refuge in the organization are encouraged to discover their talents or strengths and put them to work. People might discover those little mustard seeds from within themselves. There are many opportunities to work within the mission given that volunteers and paid staff are needed to help run the kitchen, bakery, garden, and thrift store and to keep up with office administration. In the afternoons, members of the community may gather to chop vegetables, peel potatoes, or cut butter and mix it with flour in preparation for bread making. There are also many potential sites of transference provided for people within the mission itself. There is the religious Father or the priest who acts as a support for the community. The bakery, where much funding for the organization comes from the selling of loaves to the public, provides yeast that is sometimes referred to as a "mother." There are "brothers" and "sisters" who help with the daily activities. Of course, the big Other is also present as God. The therapeutic structure of the institution manifests as an inversion of power relations where the impoverished are understood to be the masters, where people who consult with me, for instance, are also able to contribute to the labor of day-to-day operations and management of the organization. The mission's emphasis on working together helps those who have severed social bonds to reconnect. The opportunity to perform labor for the mission helps create a sense of agency and belonging for people who may not be able to easily be employed in other environments. Perhaps such labor may even help transform the symptom as a *sinthome*.

In this regard, I can supply a brief vignette. A precariously housed young person comes to mind who arrived at the mission with a court order to complete community service hours following his involvement in several robberies with a knife, the last of which ended in a stabbing and his arrest. This person spoke with me on an informal basis over coffee for many months during his time at the mission, but never developed a wish to speak with me regularly in treatment. Although I am able to regularly work with people at two or three times per week of frequency, some folks prefer to seek my ear on a more sporadic basis. Nevertheless, each time I encountered him, he had much to report, and I listened. Through working at the mission, he discovered that he could pull a knife for different purposes as he began to help the cook prepare food for meal programs. He regularly reported to me how much he enjoyed using the blades in the kitchen. This young person eventually took work elsewhere when he completed the required hours for the court as a condition of his parole. I encountered him months later on the subway. Proud and delighted, he told me that he had taken a new job as a door-to-door knife salesman! Given his previous enthusiasm for knives and taking money from people, he was already quite sharp at this job, reporting that he recently received a promotion for selling so many sets of knives. Over the course of his time at the mission, he spoke to me here and there, but found a way to support his desire outside the clinic through putting the blade to work in relation to the Other only with a little difference than before, a little twist of the knife.

Toward the Clinic

Unlike many inner-city social service agencies, the mission may be a place of busyness, but it is not so much a place of business. I find myself consistently relieved that the spiritual Fathers and clergy are more concerned with prophets and not so much with profits. In many ways, the clergy's concern for people and with only making enough to support the organization helps to facilitate the analytic situation in that there is a removal of barriers to access. There are no preconditions, no diagnoses, no assessments, no measurements, no goals, and no progress reports coming from the demand of some hyper-bureaucratic, neoliberal institutional big Other that may interfere with the direction of the treatment. The direction is towards subjectification and not objectification of the individual, but always a subjectification in relation to an Other and toward others. The referrals come directly from within the fluid community of the mission, from the clergy and staff, and from a Catholic referral service affiliated with the mission.

I hold many of the preliminary sessions over coffee or a meal in the mission before a person may decide they would like to pursue treatment. Some folks have been through so many psychiatrists and behavioral treatments that they expect I will be prescribing medications or labeling their thoughts or telling them what to do. Clinicians are rarely taught to listen anymore. Actual analytic listening is a radical gesture. As one analysand kept telling me during a consultation, "all my psychiatrist wants to do is cut me scripts." I told him I would not be "cutting his scripts" and would be listening instead, which allows me to raise a small point: scansion and the variable length session may be wonderful techniques and have a place, but I am cautious about such techniques with people who are already so used to being cut off from and by others.

You might be surprised to learn that most of my analysands do pay for their sessions. The mission subsidizes appointments, but people are asked to contribute an amount to co-pay what they can afford. This can be as little as a few dollars. As Gherovici has noted, with the minimal co-payment, analysands may regularize their attendance and become more actively involved in treatment since the symbolic payment helps to restore a sense of agency and free the analysand from building dependence and an unpayable debt ("Psychoanalysis of Poverty" 222). In the absence of payment, some analysands are already working within the mission or may take it upon themselves to wash dishes, fold laundry, sort donations, or help with other tasks so as to prevent an imaginary unpayable debt from building.

What does it mean to say that a homeless person has no address? Obviously, the person's address may be lost or precarious, but the analyst must listen to the address that comes from the body in the form of speech where the language of the subject always exceeds itself. I will conclude with a brief return to Lacan's notes at the end of his paper on "The Direction of the Treatment and the Principles of Its Power," as I hope to suggest that with the support of the mission in place, perhaps we need not stray far from these clinical recommendations when listening to the homeless subject. "Speech," writes Lacan, "possesses all the powers here, the specific powers of the treatment" (*Ecrits* 535). Unlike the Catholic or Orthodox confessional or the behavioral treatment, the analytic situation does not impose a demand that a person confesses or adapts but rather "leaves the subject free to have a go at it" (535).[8] What must be heard and seen in the mustard seed? While the subject's demands for food, shelter, and clothing may be met within the mission, the "demand is exactly what is bracketed in analysis, it being ruled out that the analyst satisfy any of the subject's demands" (535). Lacan writes that "since no obstacle is put in the way of the subject's owning of his desire, it is toward this owning that he is directed and even channeled" (535). Many analysands may say they want a home, for instance, but the resistance appears when the subject must own such a desire in being offered one, which can "be related here to nothing but desire's incompatibility with speech" (535). Of course, it has been noted in the psychoanalytic literature on attachment that homeless subjects often have difficulty with "containment" or "holding," but it surprises me that clinicians rarely consider how these signifiers carry connotations of being detained, possessed, overpowered, restrained, controlled, imprisoned, or otherwise prevented from moving freely. Many homeless people have a drive for motion, a drive to keep moving that cannot necessarily be contained. For such subjects, it may be excruciating to stay in one place if one has only known safety through dislocation, constant movement, or being outdoors. The offer of a home may be experienced as another demand from the Other. If I have not given this impression already, some analysands have trouble tolerating being in the office while speaking (at least initially) as they might feel "trapped," "suffocated," or "claustrophobic" and may prefer to leave the office door wide open or to walk or to sit outdoors on a nearby park bench while speaking with me. Lacan suggests that it will not be the analyst's "container function" that will sustain the analysand's treatment, but rather the analyst's "presence," which is "implied simply by his [or her] listening, and that this listening is simply the condition of speech. Why would analytic technique require that he make his presence so discreet if this were not, in fact, the case?" (516).[9] It is the analyst's capacity to manifest a listening presence that is most significant to reflect on in this context. I will remain uncertain if I have given you anything to take home, but if anything resonates, I hope that if you are going to provide a person living in precarious housing with a temporary hearth in your office, with a presence and not presents in the form of fulfilling the demand, that you will first have to hear the subject speak a language that is not for you.

Notes

1 This revised chapter was presented in an earlier form at the Lacan's *Écrits* Conference. Duquesne Psychology Department. Duquesne University, Pittsburgh, PA. 11–13 October 2019. A version of this revised chapter was also previously published as Vanderwees, Chris. "Dwelling on the direction of the treatment for the homeless subject." *Psychoanalytische Perspectieven*. 38.4 (2020): 411–423.

2 Even after the free clinics collapsed during the Second World War, Freud maintained hope that social responsibility toward the poor would eventually result in societies providing greater access to treatment. In a 1918 speech to the International Psychoanalytic Congress, Freud suggested that "it is possible to foresee that at some time or other the conscience of society will awake and remind it that the poor man should have just as much right to assistance for his mind as he now has to the life-saving help offered by surgery; and that the neuroses threaten public health no less than tuberculosis, and can be left as little as the latter to the impotent care of individual members of the community. When this happens, institutions or out-patient clinics will be started, to which analytically-trained physicians will be appointed, so that men who would otherwise give way to drink, women who have nearly succumbed under their burden of privations, children for whom there is no choice but between running wild or neurosis, may be made capable, by analysis, of resistance and of efficient work. Such treatments will be free. It may be a long time before the State comes to see these duties as urgent" (Freud, 1919, 167).

3 For psychoanalytic literature on homelessness and poverty, see Brown (20140; Bychowski (1970); Campbell (2006); Felix and Wine (2001); Herron and Javier (1996); Ngo-Smith, (2018); Smolen (2006); Young-Bruehl (2006).

4 For instance, Kumar overstates that "it does not take long to discern that there are virtually no writings on poverty from the French psychoanalytic tradition" (18).

5 Following Lacan and Michel Foucault (1926–1984), French clinicians including psychiatrist Jean Oury (1924–2014), psychotherapist and philosopher Felix Guattari (1930–1992), psychiatrist Frantz Fanon (1925–1961), physician Georges Canguilhem (1904–1995), and Spanish psychiatrist François Tosquelles (1912–1994) were influential thinkers within the institutional psychotherapy movement, but their work is most often applied to clinical settings that serve people suffering from psychosis rather than to a broader population of homelessness and poverty (Mackie 154–155).

6 See Hinshelwood and Manning (1979) and Manning (1989).

7 One of Kumar's primary arguments is that the psychoanalytic metaphorization of impoverishment contributes to "an inept understanding and motivation in including extra-clinical versions of reality such as chronic poverty and social adversities in the purview of psychoanalytic research and practice" (19).

8 Lacan was asked during a seminar, "Do you think that people now go to a psychoanalyst like they used to go to their confessor?" The person asking this question insists, "When you go to your analyst, you confess, too." Lacan replies to this question with his own insistence, stating a clear and important distinction between psychoanalysis and confession: "Absolutely not! They are not at all alike. In analysis, we begin by explaining to people that they are not there in order to confess. It is the first step of the art. They are there to talk – to talk about anything" (*Triumph* 63).

9 In Seminar X, Lacan writes, "Don't you know that it's not longing for the maternal breast that provokes anxiety, but its imminence? What provokes anxiety is everything that announces to us, that lets us glimpse, that we're going to be taken back to the lap. It is not, contrary to what is said, the rhythm of the mother's alternating presence and absence. The proof of this is that the infant reveals in repeating this game of presence and absence. The security of presence is the possibility of absence" (53).

Works Cited

Brown, Gabrielle. "Mothering without a home: Attachment representations and behaviours of homeless mothers and children." *Psychoanalytic Psychotherapy*. 28.4 (2014): 420–425.

Bychowski, Gustav. "Psychoanalytic reflections on the psychiatry of the poor." *The International Journal of Psychoanalysis*. 51 (1970): 503–509.

Campbell, June. "Homelessness and containment – A psychotherapy project with homeless people and workers in the homeless field." *Psychoanalytic Psychotherapy*. 20.3 (2006): 157–174.

Danto, Elizabeth Ann. *Freud's Free Clinics: Psychoanalysis & Social Justice, 1918–1938*. New York: Columbia University Press, 2005.

Felix, Alan D. and Pamela R. Wine. "From the couch to the street: Applications of psychoanalysis to work with individuals who are homeless and mentally ill." *Journal of Applied Psychoanalytic Studies*. 3.1 (2001): 17–32.

Freud, Sigmund. "Lines of Advance in Psycho-Analytic Therapy." 1919. *The Standard Edition of the Complete Psychological Works of Sigmund Freud, Volume XVII (1917–1919): An Infantile Neurosis and Other Works*. Trans. James Strachey. London: Hogarth Press, 1955.157–168.

Frosch, Allan. "Analyzability." *Psychoanalytic Review*. 93.5 (2006): 835–843.

Gherovici, Patricia. "Let's Beat Up the Poor!" *CR: The New Centennial Review*. 13.3 (2013): 1–28.

Gherovici, Patricia. "Psychoanalysis of Poverty, Poverty of Psychoanalysis." *Psychoanalysis in the Barrios*. New York: Routledge, 2019.221–235.

Herron, William G. and Rafael A. Javier. "The psychogenesis of poverty: Some psycho analytic conceptions." *The Psychoanalytic Review*. 83.4 (1996): 611–620.

Hinshelwood, Robert and Nick Manning (eds). *Therapeutic Communities: Reflections and Progress*. London: Routledge, 1979.

Kumar, Manasi. "The poverty in psychoanalysis: 'Poverty' of psychoanalysis." *Psychology and the Developing Societies*. 24 (2012): 1–34.

Lacan, Jacques. *Écrits: The First Complete Edition in English*. 1966. Trans. Bruce Fink. New York: W.W. Norton & Co, 2006.

Lacan, Jacques. "The Direction of the Treatment and the Principles of Its Power." *Écrits: The First Complete Edition in English*. 1966. Trans. Bruce Fink. New York: W.W. Norton & Co, 1958/2006. 489–542.

Lacan, Jacques. *The Seminar of Jacques Lacan, Book X: Anxiety*. 2004. Trans. A.R. Price. Ed. Jacques-Alain Miller. New York: Polity Press, 2014.

Lacan, Jacques. *The Triumph of Religion Preceded by Discourse to Catholics*. 2005. Trans. Bruce Fink. New York: Polity Press, 2013.

Mackie, Brenda. *Treating People with Psychosis in Institutions: A Psychoanalytic Perspective*. London: Karnac, 2016.

Manning, Nick. *The Therapeutic Community Movement: Charisma and Routinization*. Routledge: New York, 1989.

Ngo-Smith, Brian R. "This couch has bedbugs: On the psychoanalysis of homelessness in the homelessness of psychoanalysis." *Clinical Social Work*. 46 (2018): 26–33.

Smolen, Ann G. "'Home is where one starts from': An Analysis of a Homeless Child." *Fort Da*. 12.1 (2006): 42–61.

St. John the Compassionate Mission. *To Give a Beautiful Witness: The Rule of St. John the Compassionate*. Toronto: St. John the Compassionate Mission, 2016.

Young-Bruehl, Elizabeth. "Coming of age in New York City: Two homeless boys." *The Psychoanalytic Quarterly*. 75.1 (2006): 323–343.

Chapter 5

Psychoanalysis is Spoken Here

Analytic Ethics and the Talking Cure in the Delivery of Community Mental Health Treatment

Christopher Meyer

> So, I believe that the future of analysis in this country does not lie with the medical establishment. It lies with the people of the universities, with you ladies and gentlemen; especially, I would say, with young people not yet established in a career and who are now keen on putting Lacan's teaching to use. . . . In so far as some among them, at least will in the long run have sufficient belief in what they themselves think concerning psychoanalysis to enter analytic experience proper and perhaps (for some of them at least) to practice it, it is they, the new analysts stemming from the universities (and some, I hope from the medical profession) who could in time change the course of American psychoanalysis.
>
> (Miller, 1991, 84–85)

Jacques-Alain Miller's words – addressed at a conference held at Kent State in 1988 whose keynote speakers were subsequently published in a collection of essays entitled *Lacan and the Subject of Language* – struck me as a good place to begin a consideration of where psychoanalysis stands in its relationship to the delivery of community mental health treatment in the 21st century. Reading them today, and knowing they were spoken before they were written, I read Miller's words as a call to the analyst of the future and to the possibilities of a future for psychoanalysis as a clinical practice that contests the history of psychoanalysis as it has been established in the United States. Throughout his life, Lacan called for a return to Freud, or a return to the logic and experience of the rupture Freud's invention confronts us with as human or speaking beings. Lacan's return to Freud directs us to the inception of the analytic experience and re-orients us to the central place that desire, the Other's desire, takes in the emergence of the unconscious in the analytic experience at the time of its infancy, a time and an experience we refer to Freud's name as its father. Lacan's call also refers us to Lacan's name as a signifier articulating a savoir, or knowledge, that orients us towards the logical trajectory of an analytic experience, especially as regards its termination in the object

DOI: 10.4324/9781003212072-6

of the fundamental fantasy and the insistence of a *jouissance* beyond the phallus.

As a call, Miller offers no prescription or guidance as to how a future for psychoanalysis in the United States will come to pass. His remarks fall, rather, in the logical place of desire, an Other's desire, and function in a way that is not entirely dissimilar to the very advent of the human or speaking being insofar as its experience begins with the effraction of the voice, first object cause of desire, and material support of the signifier as its Other hooks that thing at work in each one of us to the signifiers selected in the inscription of its excess. But it was not just Miller who came calling at this conference. I cite his words in order to mark an uncanny sense of time as regards the time it has taken for the practice of Freudian–Lacanian psychoanalysis to take hold clinically in the United States, which is only in its infancy when psychoanalysis is understood as taking place in the aftermath of Lacan's return to Freud.

Along with Miller's talk, Willy Apollon's essay (Apollon, 1991) on the treatment of psychosis at the 388, a clinic for young adult psychotics in Québec City, stands out insofar as it points to the ways in which psychoanalysis is reinvented in community mental health and makes a space for the unconscious of the underserved and society's most marginalized. Apollon's essay clearly links this to psychoanalytic ethics whose point of orientation is to make way for the speech of subjects who are historically at the margins of society and treatment and deemed at or beyond the limit of its scope of practice by traditional approaches to psychoanalysis. Apollon's essay introduces us to a paradigmatic shift that takes place in the experience and theory of the psychoanalytic clinic when psychosis is given a place to be heard. Psychoanalysis goes further when it is able to welcome and learn from those whose speech was heretofore on its margins, unwelcomed by the analyst, or even seen as "untreatable" by it. A reading of early Freud reminds us that psychoanalysis is possible and arises at the limit between that which can be treated and that which is untreatable, and it is precisely because the analysts of GIFRIC have worked on that line or margin that psychoanalysis is pushed further as a clinical practice. The psychotic's experience re-orients us to the central place of unconscious formations for creating a space for the subject and, as Alfredo Carrasquillo has argued, a "repositioning of the person with psychosis" (Carrasquillo, 94, 2019). The dream becomes the royal road for not just the unconscious but also the possibility of giving a position to the subject and a space or gap between the subject and the discourse of the delusion where the tyranny of the *jouissance* of the Other reigns. Carrasquillo writes that "an individual who has been freed from the insurmountable demands of an imaginary other, . . . , is an individual with social and political agency, a citizen among other citizens" (Carrasquillo, 2019). Their work with psychotics has resulted in a mutation in the concept and experience of transference and the ethics of the psychoanalyst as regards the unconscious knowledge at work in that subjective structure.

The ethical position of the analyst called for in Apollon's work regards the relationship between a given community and the psychoanalytic clinic that serves it and challenges us to rethink the psychoanalytic clinic as one that meets the community where and as it is in order to create a space for the knowledge or savoir at work there to have its say. What is unique about psychoanalysis in the aftermath of Lacan are the ways in which the analyst's offer of a lack in knowing is the only guarantee of constituting the analytic experience or discourse. At the level of practice, this means that in the psychoanalytic clinic the analyst's stance is one that does not offer or apply a treatment to those it has historically deemed untreatable; rather, psychoanalysis is pushed further when its treatment is constructed from and based upon listening to the speech and experience of those it serves and is oriented by the untreatable at work in them. Grounded as it is in a social link in which the Other of the address is absent, psychoanalytic ethics and practice are uniquely positioned for welcoming such speech.

Miller very clearly differentiates a future for psychoanalysis "in this country" as one that makes its way into the experience and practice of the clinic through the university where Lacan is "used" in the study of literature, film, art history and theory, etc. He goes on to declare his hope that those who use it will in turn be *used* by it, given that it is the unconscious that uses us and not the other way around. To think about this future from the perspective of Lacan's discourse theory, the hope is that the very thing at work in them as students at the university in their study of Lacan and Freud will constitute a symptom whose insistence will lead them to the door of an analyst, and that after much work in their personal analysis, they in turn will adopt the position of the analyst in clinical practice. This adoption in turn welcomes the arrival of the one who makes the demand for an analytic experience.

Just because Lacan is smuggled into the United States through the university does not guarantee results at the level of the clinic. It is the analytic experience and not its theory that creates mutations in the social link. But it is important to acknowledge how Lacan's return to Freud arrived and made its impact here in the United States, where the ground was seeded and irrigated in departments of critical theory, art history, comparative literature, cultural studies, and film studies for what would result in psychoanalytic clinical practice. Freud's advocacy of a "lay analysis" looked to the study of literature, philosophy, mathematics, sociology, and anthropology as the way forward for the plague he brought to the shores of the United States, only to find it seized at entry by the medical establishment. That seizure of a discursive praxis was due to the radical unseating of the autonomy of the ego inaugurated by the Freudian rupture at the beginning of the 20th century. It was a rupture antithetical to what Lacan and Freud would both see as the

American way of life, where a devotion to the relentless gaze of the almighty dollar forms the currency of the capitalist discourse. Lacan's return to Freud is what Miller is talking about in his call because Lacan himself placed his bet on Freud's name as a point of orientation for thinking about what is at stake in the psychoanalytic clinic. This seizure of psychoanalysis has been so effective in its institution in the United States where Lacan is *not* spoken, that the psychoanalytic institutes – suddenly awakened to questions of social justice, equity of access, and the importance of cultural considerations raised in the wake of the George Floyd murder – find themselves resorting to an effort to "rebrand" psychoanalysis. To "rebrand" psychoanalysis is the explicit language used by one of the more prominent psychoanalytic institutes here in Los Angeles. This response to calls for equity, inclusion, and discussions on culture and race in the psychoanalytic institute is a long overdue reckoning with the ways in which the institution of psychoanalysis in the United States has drifted ever further from its imbrication in questions regarding culture, class, race, and social justice, which arise from the given of its experience – that the unconscious is structured by and like a language where norms, ideals, prohibitions, and factor C, or culture, constitute the ego's discourse in which the subject of the unconscious is embedded (on "factor C" cf. Lacan, 2006b, 264; Apollon, 1997, 48–50). As part of this enterprise to rebrand and hence to reassert its relevance in the 21st century, the psychoanalytic establishment implicates itself in the discourse of capitalism and the marketplace, and forgets Elizabeth Danto's reminder in her seminal work on Freud's *Free Clinics, Psychoanalysis and Social Justice, 1918–1938* – that Freud's dream of "free clinics" as a form of social justice had a history throughout Europe that arose in the aftermath of the first world war. They also seem to have no awareness of the aliveness of psychoanalysis in the community mental health clinic outside the United States, in countries where Lacan's return to Freud continues to see the practitioner's responsibility as one of hewing to the unconscious, and sees psychoanalysis as a practice in which the Other, rather than the ego, self, or person, is given a frame in which to be heard through its formations. For those of us whose work and formation take place with reference to Freud and Lacan, there is no need for rebranding, or renaming: we have only to install the remainder of what was set to work in us at the end of our analysis and create clinical spaces where speech is given a frame for the work of the unconscious.

What's in a Name, or Nomination Is Not Rebranding

Just eight years prior to the conference where Miller and Apollon spoke, Lacan was still alive and giving a seminar in Caracas, Venezuela, referred to as the seminar "Dissolution." As he spoke about his School and its "cause freudienne," Lacan would create a sort of trait d'union between his name and Freud's for those practicing in the aftermath of his teaching when he said, "It is for you to call yourselves Lacanian, as for me, I am Freudian." And although he would go on to clarify how his introduction of the topological registers of the Real, Symbolic, and the Imaginary introduce a "three" different from Freud's three of the Oedipus myth, by placing Freud in the place of "cause," Lacan would go on in his seminar on dissolution to underscore the degree to which what those of us after Lacan refer to as the letters of the body at work in the so-called Real unconscious owe their "cause" to Freud's other myth – that of the drive. In the field of the drive, freed of the imaginary Other of seduction, Lacan's work points the way to thinking through the experience of castration beyond Oedipus and beyond the symbolic father as a point of orientation. Another kind of call is at stake here, then, that concerns how we call and name ourselves as analysts in the wake of Lacan's return to Freud, and not as "Lacanians or Freudians," but rather as analysts whose ethic is oriented by the hole in language that constitutes the rupture speech makes in its first call to the object that falls from the voice.

The self-nomination of the analyst is one of the anti-institutional turns of Lacan's teaching. But there is something more at stake in this question of naming, self-nomination, and in whose name one positions one's act and one's reinvention of psychoanalysis in the becoming-analyst. By making such a claim regarding his own name, and by referring himself to the name of the father of psychoanalysis, Lacan confronts today's psychoanalysts who return to Freud with that question of how to create new spaces within the social link, *clinical spaces*. Returning to Freud calls for a response in the being of the clinician and a capacity to act from what is set to work in them by the rupture the unconscious makes in their being. The analytic clinic is a space for the speech act insofar as when a patient asks for an analysis, the analyst-to-be faces a choice: to act from the position of the analyst whose only guarantee is the lack and the object at work there, or to provide a therapy to the ego. At the level of the clinic, the consequences of what position the clinician takes when faced with the question of receiving the request for analysis is consequential and determinative insofar as the response and responsibility of the analyst is to make space for what could not otherwise be heard or spoken by the subject of the unconscious and what will and cannot be heard if the act of the clinician is one that offers a treatment to the ego. There is an ask and there is an act, and it is to act from that object (object cause of desire, oriented by that *cause freudienne*) set to work in them to the request their patients make to them for analytic treatment, and to which they respond with a specific offer – the offer of an analytic experience – that makes speech possible in the face of the Other's desire and call.

Having received that call myself some years ago, and having spent some time in my own psychoanalytic formation, as an analyst supervising and practicing in community mental health clinics, and in private practice, I have come to the conclusion that what we face in the United States today concerns seeing to it that psychoanalysis is spoken in community mental health clinics and, for those of us who have been working in such spaces, to account for the results of our work. It is only by taking these results into account, and by drawing from our experience at the level of the clinic, that those of us who adhere to this social bond can think about how we can push that work further in order to supply an analytic response to the demands and, even more importantly, the desire of the subjects of the 21st century for that which is at work in them and which science, civilization, the marketplace, and medical and therapeutic approaches exclude. These latter are ever more organized around a model of consumerism in which the product or outcome is determinative and acts as an answer to the lack or defect in the Other of the address. They cannot tolerate the anxiety that comes from supporting a question that engages the subject in a singular creativity arising in the environs of the hole, lack, and absence of the Other that is the a priori in the experience of the human or speaking being. Because of its position with regard to what cannot and will not be said to an Other who supplies a prefabricated answer or treatment, psychoanalysis creates an opening for the singular creativity at work in its user's discontents.

Of First and Last Calls

I first read Miller's essay in 1992, and it was at or around that same time that three analysts from Québec City were invited to the University of California, Irvine, to give several lectures on the ethics of femininity and their work with young adult psychotics at their clinic, known as the 388. Like a few of my fellow graduate students who were in the audience that weekend, we were well immersed in the intersections of comparative literature, critical theory, and psychoanalysis. But none of us could have foreseen what was being set to work in us by what we heard there and then in the University Club where we sat and listened. In psychoanalysis, it is the desire-to-know of the analyst that calls the subject forth. The patient's encounter with the analyst's desire-to-know lays the conditions of possibility for transference to the unconscious, which thereby overturns the Other of seduction and care. In what I am calling transference, the patient makes a symbolic move from one of receiving care to one of becoming an analysand, or the one who assumes a love for the knowledge that comes from the unconscious – the unconscious as an Other place – to which they are subject. This knowledge is constituted and elaborated through the signifiers selected by the letters of the body, regarding the impasse between the knowledge constructed in the chaining of signifiers (S2) and the truth of the subject (S1) that holds onto the Real as always only ever half-spoken, mi-dire for Lacan, or unreceivable by any Other.

It would be some years later, after having read the articles by Miller and Apollon cited above and after having entered into my own analytic formation, that I found myself beginning a lengthy apprenticeship in community mental health settings where psychoanalysis was tolerated but not the lingua franca. And it was in one of those (dis)placements, while working at a methadone clinic that I would find myself receiving my instructions from my supervisor about my position as a "counselor." I would have a caseload of 50 clients, a great deal of freedom regarding the frequency and length of session, and he said something that has always stayed with me: "for many of our clients this is their last call." This, in addition to the fact that the clinic's approach to substance abuse treatment was grounded in harm reduction and motivational interviewing, made it possible to enter the room with no specific agenda or treatment protocol to apply when meeting with my clients. Every session was oriented by a basic question that, whether spoken or not, took the form of an invitation: "what do you want to do with this time of speech?" As a time for speech, the counseling session transcended the question of what the "dose," or what the clinic as Other, held and distributed to them. As I look back in retrospect and consider this question of time in its relationship to first as well as last calls, and given a certain being-towards-death that was more often than not inscribed in the numerous co-occurring issues at work in the bodies of the underserved and marginalized persons who made up my caseload this question of speech, and the importance of supporting its occasion on my side, feels all the more pressing.

I quickly learned there were two separate spaces in the clinic – one upstairs and one downstairs – each of which constituted separate yet importantly interconnected symbolic spaces. As a clinician, I awaited the arrival of my clients upstairs except in the exceptional circumstances in which ambulatory considerations prohibited them from negotiating the stairs. For these, I reserved a room below. Upstairs was a place for speech, for the talking cure, whereas downstairs was where the clinic's patients received their dose of methadone, and where the medical director had her office. The field of the gaze was fully operational downstairs, where the nursing staff would scan and assess the relative sobriety of the person receiving their dose, check in with them with small talk, and then ask them to take a breathalyzer prior to receiving their guava-juice colored dose. It was also downstairs where blood was drawn and viral loads of Hep C were tracked for those undergoing treatment for their liver condition. Upstairs was where people came to speak about any and everything going on in their lives, including how things were going in their "opioid replacement therapy" taking place downstairs.

Each One is Subject to an Other to Whom the Analyst Makes a Call

What I discovered working upstairs is that the analyst's desire places its call in the Other, the Other to which the analysand is subject, and the response of this Other is guaranteed by one thing and one thing only: that this call from the analyst entails an act that stems from a desire-to-know rather than a knowledge. This is an important distinction in the psychoanalytic clinic in that its aim is to make space for the unconscious, or what Freud called an Other scene/eine andere Schauplatz in his *Interpretation of Dreams* (Freud, 536). For Freud, the idea of such an other scene suggests a psychical topology, or a psychical locality, other than the ego or expression of self in everyday life. If psychoanalysis is to be spoken in the community mental health clinic, as my title suggests, doing so makes space for this scene of the Other, whose expression takes the form of the unconscious formations of the dream, bungled actions, slips of the tongue and witticisms, daydreams, symptoms, and the act where it becomes visible. In the field of neurosis, the unconscious shows up as a rupture that contests the discourse of the ego and its montage of seduction, which is grounded in the demand for love and hate from the Other. The subject of the signifier appears as a flash or a sudden revelation where speech fails and founders in the domain of the unspeakable, and it is precisely where the signifier fails to say it all regarding this one, this Other, to whom the speaking being is subject, that the rupture of the Other scene registers and works its way into the experience of the client. And although any chance of the Other being flushed out from the bush arises from the speech of the client, the position taken by the clinician in relation to their speech either welcomes or silences the possibility of the Other's arrival into the treatment.

Any possibility of hearing from the Other to whom the client or patient is subject(ed), any chance to hear from the language system with all of its intersectional dynamics, is guaranteed by the lack the analyst offers the patient who is called to become an analysand. The nature of this speech-act and how to take responsibility for the effects of the analytic act as well as the degree to which the object at work in the analyst solicits speech from the subject is what is learned in so-called Control, or the supervision of the Candidate-Analyst in training. Control is the experience in the Lacanian School through which the clinician, or Candidate-Analyst, takes responsibility for having said yes to the request for a psychoanalysis from the client. Lacan had many definitions for what "makes" the analyst, and he was well aware of the possibility of imposture as well as the lures towards mastery that "being an analyst" entails. But beyond the so-called self-authorization of the analyst, Lacan's observation that it is the analysand that *makes* the analyst brings us to the heart of the ethical stakes for the one who assumes responsibility for the position of analyst and for the object that "acts" to create a space for the unconscious in the clinical experience.

For the clinician to make such a call is simply to give the patient a chance – a chance to experience the particularity of their desire and to have a place to speak of it, to find the words that give way to speech that concerns the rupture the Other scene, or the unconscious, has made in their lives, and to have a place to work from that. The analyst's desire-to-know serves as a call that makes space for both an Other and its subject. The clinician therefore makes an "offer," as Willy Apollon will argue, that "always places the human experience at the heart of every clinical perspective as a positivity from which it is necessary to set out" (Apollon, 1999, 18). This positivity brings us to the heart of what Apollon defines as the "untreatable" in more recent writings (Apollon, 2006). An analytic clinic conceived with such a positivity in mind, where that thing set to work in the speaking being by the effractions of the voice makes in the logic and being of the human calls for a new position in relation to the symptom by both analysand and analyst. Rather than view the symptom as a disorder, defect, or even foreclosure to be treated or corrected, the analyst welcomes the symptom as a path towards the object that functions as the very cause of the desire to live, work, and create something new for humanity. Such a "positivity" takes us to the heart of a "specificity" and a singularity in the subject's relation to the Other. Apollon writes from the perspective of over 40 years working with psychosis, but as those listed on my caseload walked through the door, my offer was oriented by the very positivity of their experience and their suffering insofar as it was seeking a place to be heard. However simple this may sound, it is in fact all too rare in the community mental health clinic and requires a specific offer and position from the clinician that is grounded in analytic ethics as regards speech and desire. My position was tolerated upstairs in the clinic where I worked, but the analytic act and position I assumed there did not form the basis for the clinic's paradigm for thinking about opioid dependency and addiction.

From Addiction to (*a*) Diction, *Infans*, and the Rupture of the Unconscious

I have written elsewhere of the opening move made by the unconscious in an analytic treatment with an analysand, M, who was a patient in a methadone clinic (Meyer, 2011). In that case, the Other that first made the scene in M's speech took the form of a bungled action. This unconscious formation opened a space for hearing something beyond the preoccupation with raising his dose of methadone to an "ideal dose" that would help him manage the pain he felt in his neck and back, a pain he also linked to what he saw as his difficulties losing weight. Beyond the presenting symptom and demand evoked in his speech about wanting to lose weight and a desire to achieve an "ideal dose," M's bungled action took us to an Other scene where his desire was playing itself out in relations with his ex-wife, his mother, and finally, as later sessions would reveal, the recollection of a man who molested him as an adolescent.

In his first session, it was as M drifted into the stream of his associations forming the day – residue of his annoyance fending off the unwanted flirtation of an older woman at a party and after he worked on associations to having left the keys to his wife's house with the analyst (the bungled action) – that his work on the dream yielded the following formulation: "get this woman off my back." This phrase, a demand beyond the immediate demand of wanting to reach his "ideal" dose and weight, would articulate the letter of the body where *jouissance* had inscribed itself throughout his subjective history – his neck and back – and allow him to create space between the *jouissance* of an Other (his mother) who in his fantasy had "killed his father" and with whom he found himself "trapped" in the aftermath of his father's death when, as a child, he encountered her voice emerging from the bedroom where she slowly drank herself to death. He had taken "the woman" on his back, and it was only as he realized in freeing himself from the expectation of receiving financial support from his ex-wife and coming to terms with the binds of the imaginary debt he had incurred that M was able to return to his creative projects and support himself again through his music and art.

As a working hypothesis, I suggest that my choice to ask M about his dreams and his bungled action – his leaving the keys in my office belonging to his ex-wife who had asked him to return them – functioned as a response from M's unconscious to the analyst's act. In other words, it was because I spoke of my desire to hear from his unconscious as I established the frame at the very beginning of the treatment that M's unconscious gave an answer. I am well aware of the metric called for to demonstrate progress in treatment in evidence-based treatment approaches and that my hypothesis falls outside of the range of such a metric. But I am equally aware that the metric for evidence in the analytic experience differs from what is demanded of the practitioner in the so-called evidence-based approaches. In psychoanalysis, evidence and the evidential concern the response from the unconscious of the analysand and an awaiting of the movement of transference on the part of the analysand, which involves a shift in their ethical position as a subject in relation to the suffering at work in the symptom. The symptom must have its say. It does so by finding key words, or signifiers, that articulate the subject in his or her relationship to the fantasies that constitute their experience of the Other to whom they are subject. Work on the symptom takes place in the clinic of fantasy where the Other of the primal scene fantasy insists, and the Other of the seduction fantasy (in neurosis) falls. The fall of the Other opens a space to the fantasy of castration where, supported by the phallus, defined as the signifier of the Other's desire, the subject assumes the lack and absence of any Other capable of receiving their truth or providing satisfaction to the excess at work in them. The experience of castration is an experience of the singular ways in which a given subject takes responsibility for their desire and forms part of the time and field in the termination phase of the analytic experience – the time when the object of the fundamental fantasy is constructed to remain as the signature of the subject in the assumption of desire and *jouissance* in a new space in the social link. To stick with the unconscious formation alone, a certain undecidability is always at work as regards the cause of a dream (its day residue), a symptom, a slip of the tongue, a joke or witticism, "failed" or bungled act, or act of the unconscious. The unconscious formation alone serves as evidence, and the work regarding its cause is approached through fantasy. To assume the desire at work in it as well as a capacity to take responsibility for the excess or *jouissance* at work there, heavy lifting is required on the part of the analysand in the construction of the unknown, or unconscious, knowing that it is at work in the presenting complaint or symptom.

It is with his introduction of the object (a) as cause of desire, and with the voice as a rupture in the experience of the speaking being, that Lacan and those working in his aftermath confront us with the necessity of making a space for the clinic of fantasy regarding that first object, what Apollon refers to as a solely mental representation in his essay on "The Untreatable," that falls from the voice and constitutes the destiny of the speaking being as subject. The clinic of fantasy is one in which the work of analysis concerns four logical moments in the experience of the subject. These are: the primal scene or originary fantasy (a fantasy of being subjected to the *jouissance* of the Other and thereby obliterated as subject of desire), the seduction fantasy (the resort in neurosis to being loved, hated, and ultimately spared from the *jouissance* of the Other in which the death of the subject is inscribed), the castration fantasy, or that fantasy of the body's separation from the organism that delivers the being over to the work of the signifier in its relation to the excess introduced by it as well as to the failure or defect in the signifier to represent the subject in their relation to desire and *jouissance*, and finally, to the clinic of the fundamental fantasy, or the construction of that remainder, that object cause that continues to insist in the desire and *jouissance* of the divided or barred subject.

As regards the possibility of becoming well spoken about the object (a) at stake in the analytic experience, I want to emphasize how the speaking being's subjection to speech and language results in something essential in humanity, which is well articulated by the concept of castration Lacan introduces in *Seminar V* when he speaks of the "final fantasy" in the three fantasies that constitute Freud's essay, "A Child Is Being Beaten." What is essential for Lacan and for psychoanalysis is the experience of castration, or the ways in which the speaking being is subject to speech and language or, more fundamentally, to the Other of the address in the articulation of its needs, demands, and desires. This subjection to the Other – an Other that exists as an absence, is at stake and put into play in any appeal for help made to the practitioner working in our systems of care. The Other precedes the subject, and the experience of being subject to the Other is constitutive of the field of speech and language, the field of the unconscious, and must be taken into consideration whenever a psychoanalytic approach is at work. As Lacan writes:

> human beings, as such, are all under the stick. To enter into the world of desire is for the human being to undergo, right at the outset, the law imposed by this something that exists beyond – that we were calling the law of the father is no longer of any importance, it doesn't matter – the law of the rod. This is how, for a determinate subject entering the matter by particular pathways, a certain line of evolution is defined.
>
> (Lacan, 2017, 226)

In the psychoanalytic clinic, the "world of desire" insists "right at the outset." It is a world that points beyond the law of the father to the "law of the rod," the rod of speech and language that cut the speaking being off from immediate and total satisfaction and deliver him or her over to another logic – the logic of desire and the excess at work in the body of the one who is subject to the address to the Other. The function of this cut, this castration, is to deliver the speaking being over to a field beyond the law and beyond Oedipus. The speaking being is delivered to a life, a space, and a time that is oriented by the object cause of desire and will discover the signifiers that support him in this quest. We are always working with this *before*- and *after*-birth insofar as, at the level of the clinic, the analytic experience concerns a subject whose fall into being sets off from an encounter with the rupture made by the voice of the Other, whose logic and particular pathways will be elaborated during the course of the analytic experience. To stay within the field of addiction and to move towards an ethic of the well spoken, or (a) diction: this is what I will turn to now as we consider the ways in which the future Freudian and Lacanian clinic can create spaces in which something essential – the unreceivable – to the experience of the speaking being can be welcomed and worked on in the frame of the treatment.

The work of another analysand orients us to the ethics required of a speech that traverses or passes through the Other whose absence the analyst supports. The traversal transcends the shortcut of addiction, whose demand for cure conforms to the logic of the marketplace and capitalism where the Other in the socio-economic system is "holding" the object, or gadget, that promises to satisfy the speaker. It is when we listen to the testimonies of those veterans who have survived their personal war on drugs, in the clinic as well as in the literature of addiction, that we can begin to fathom the degree to which the product degrades the customer when it comes to the marketplace and its promise of full-service satisfaction. As a social link that depends upon and guarantees the lack in the Other of the address, the analytic clinic constrains the analysand to encounter the lack, thereby reactivating the drive and the excess that has been encoded in the symptom whose "sense," or fantasy, will be constructed in the course of the treatment

(Freud, 1917, 257–272). Such a construction is not in itself a cure and departs from the popular notion of rendering the unconscious conscious that forms the typical formulation of psychoanalytic and psycho-dynamic treatment approaches. Instead, the construction of a new knowledge regarding the object of fantasy confronts the subject with an ethical choice regarding their enjoyment and investment in the symptom, and a new position with regard to the symptom as an expression of what could not otherwise be spoken. The analysand comes to find in the symptom a cipher for an unspeakable Real seeking its way into speech beyond any Other capable of receiving or silencing it.

Rather than an obstacle to be removed, the symptom is taken up as the pathway of a Real where things don't work out in the life of the speaking being, but where desire and drive are at work. The symptom therefore points us in the direction of what goes to the very core of what is worth living and dying for. The traversal of the symptom in the clinic of the fantasy therefore confronts the subject with the possibility and challenge of bringing something new to humanity – something that is caused by that first object whose (a)topia requires more (more speech, more work, and more acts) of the subject of desire to give it space and time in the social link.

Speech and the Body: An Inaugural Dream, or "I Keep My Power in the Bag"

By the time he arrived for analysis, W had already encountered several systems of care and was engaged in the self-help groups of Narcotics Anonymous and Alcoholics Anonymous. A 30-day hospitalization several years before calling the analyst, ongoing involvement with a sponsor in his self-help group, and numerous therapies, each one of which he described as having arrived at a familiar impasse regarding what could not be said in the face of what he calculated the other wanted for and from him – all of these efforts at recovery preceded his decision to begin an analysis. He spoke of wanting to take the risk of beginning an analysis. He first took a real interest in psychoanalysis when he chose Freud's "Thoughts for the Times on War and Death" as his assignment for a high school rhetoric course some 15 years prior to appearing at the analyst's door. Having been sober now for almost five years, his presenting complaint in his most recent therapy with a Dr. P, whose name he made into a witticism by speaking of him as Dr. Purse, concerned a dysfunctional relationship with a girlfriend he had spent the past year trying unsuccessfully to break up with. He reported having cut himself off from family and friends as he delved into this intoxicating relationship, said he was stalled in his career, but he had not cut himself off from the family purse, which had paid for his treatment with his former therapist, "Dr. Purse." He may have cut himself off from heroin, but he could not leave the heroine. And the purse itself was a point of reference as he recalled having wanted to be a thief as a child of 5 or 6, and remembered how he would "steal my father's money from my mother's purse" and bury it in the backyard, where he kept his treasure buried in the sandbox. This, along with his mother's admonitions that he "hid his light in a bushel" and a series of other associations, rendered the joke made at the expense of his former therapist rich with irony regarding his sense of having kept his hand in the "purse" and bag of the mother for far too long.

He experienced some immediate relief in his preliminary sessions when he discovered, through the phonemic play of an alphabetic letter, that he found himself caught in a displacement from heroin to the heroine, and he began to question what he was pursuing in the relationship he could not quit. Several events came together to form the day residue of an inaugural dream that would serve as a reference point in the years of analysis that followed: he was looking for a new apartment and was therefore "homeless," and he had finally broken things off with his heroine after she had "kicked him out of her home." In the dream:

> a harmless homeless man approaches carrying a large plastic bag. He says, "What I've got in the bag is real powerful," and "I keep my power in the bag." He then says in a pleasant tone and as a statement of fact, "I just might hit you." I and an other . . . leave the canyon by a short cut. My pocket watch falls to the canyon floor and I say I will return for it later. As I am leaving the canyon my mother tells me the best way back to the canyon is by way of Pebble Beach Mall.

The dream takes us to the heart of the question of the Other of the address as one who is or is not holding something "real powerful" in the bag, and it also indicates where power is held – in this bag. The dream is itself an interpretation of a Real encountered by the analysand in his daily life (day residue). As the analysis proceeds, the key signifiers of the dream ("hit," "power," "bag," as well as the time-piece and the canyon) link the subject to a *jouissance* representing the barred subject as subject to a Real and thus a beyond, to what Lacan referred to as the semblance of the signifier. These signifiers will continue to insist as the analysand "returns later" to this dream in the course of his analysis.

The dream is a transference dream insofar as he associates the "harmless homeless man" with the analyst who was at that time in the process of moving his office. The analyst was also"homeless." But the dream also ushers in a transference beyond the person of the analyst, or this Other who "just might hit you" and who "keeps his power in the bag." The dream itself becomes an object of transference as further material unpacks the content of the "bag," revealing signifiers linked to letters of the body and repetitive symptoms that had plagued him throughout his life. Being in the bag was also to be strung out on black tar heroin, sold on the street in bags or balloons, and in pursuit of which he spent much time and money – never to be returned.

In addition to the analyst, we have the mother, who indicates the "best way back to the canyon" into which his pocket watch has fallen – a place into which, as the analysand associates, he "loses time," and which is linked to a childhood trauma and memory of a visit he made with his family to a canyon that makes him think of "shit" – the "canyon of shit." The question of time concerns something left in the bag, something to return to, and will be linked in a later phase of the analysis to the effraction made by the voice of the father, who had expressed his concern that his son suffered from a "failure to thrive." Along the course of the treatment, he would find more words to evoke the power discovered and enjoyed in the bag of the m(O)ther as well as the ways in which desire was discovered beyond her. That way pointed to the realization he must "fail her to thrive," and to the construction of an object that had no currency in the purse of his mother filled with his father's coins. That realm, the realm beyond the Other of seduction and beyond the father he so loved and hated would lead to an "out house" of desire and excess where new words could be found and new works created. What called for a "failing her" to thrive revealed something that would always be in the bag, *infans*, that had not found a way to speak but that later dreams and unconscious formations would deliver.

There is neither space nor time in this essay to track the various chains of the signifier and their link to the inscription of *jouissance* in the letters of the body, their encoding in the symptom, and finally, the failure and defect of the signifier encircling the construction of the object of the fundamental fantasy as they relate retroactively to this dream. Doing so is part of a longer project that aims at pushing ever further into the very possibility of speech that concerns the object cause of desire, which is the object in the analytic experience. This pursuit forms part of the ethics of the well spoken, or (a) diction, called for in the transmission of psychoanalysis in the psychoanalytic school after Lacan. The possibility of becoming ever more well spoken about the clinic of fantasy and the logical term of the analytic experience is just one of the many crucial problems that remain to be addressed, as those who return to Freud's desire through Lacan's savoir say more about the analytic experience and create more spaces that are embedded within their respective communities and cultures, so that what is at work and at stake in the speaking being can be articulated and assumed by the subject.

Psychoanalysis is a practice whose conditions of possibility depend upon the capacity to construct an address for the unspeakable. Given the demands placed upon beginning practitioners to adhere to and to apply evidence-based treatment to the suffering and discontents of speaking beings, it is important to raise and pursue the question of what place psychoanalysis has in the delivery of community mental health treatment, insofar as the ethics of the psychoanalyst's act is to make space within the analytic frame for that which is both unspeakable and untreatable in the life of the speaking, or human, being. An ethical stance is called for – a stance grounded in psychoanalytic ethics – in order to hold a space for work with, from, and on the unconscious in the community mental health clinic with individuals identified as experiencing "severity" – in the fields of addiction, the psychoses, and the so-called borderline states. Far from being unresponsive to or beyond the scope of analytic practice, psychoanalysis holds a space for the subject of the unconscious, even in the face of severity. Returning to Freud's dream of "free clinics," psychoanalysis practiced after Lacan creates space for the subject of our time to be heard. As an experience and a social link, psychoanalysis aims beyond the worried well, taking us to the heart of the discontents of civilization. And it is solely on the basis of its adherence to unconscious formations that a path can be forged to a subject's "truth" regarding what would necessarily remain unsaid, repressed, and radically censored. In this adherence, the analytic act aims for the evocation and constitution of a new position taken by the analysand in their relationship to their presenting complaint and to the cause underlying their symptom and suffering.

Works Cited

Apollon, W. (1991). Theory and practice in the psychoanalytic treatment of psychosis. In *Lacan and the Subject of Language* (pp. 116–140). New York: Routledge.

Apollon, W. (1997). Du spécifique à l'Universel entre sens et contresens. In *L'Universel, perspectives psychanalytiques* (pp. 37–50). Québec, Canada: Gifric.

Apollon, W. (1999). *Psychoses: l'offre de l'analyste*. Québec, Canada: Gifric.

Apollon, W. (2006). The untreatable. *Umbr(a), A Journal of the Unconscious*: 23–39.

Carrasquillo, A. (2019). The anxiety of citizenship, or the psychotic as citizen. In *Psychoanalysis in the Barrios* (pp. 87–96). New York: Routledge.

Danto, Elizabeth. (2005). *Freud's Free Clinics: Psychoanalysis and Social Justice, 1918–1938*. New York: Columbia University Press.

Freud, S. (1900). The Interpretation of Dreams (Second Part). In J. Strachey (Ed.), *The Standard Edition of the Complete Psychological Works of Sigmund Freud, Volume V (1900–1901)*. London, England: Hogarth Press.

Freud, S. (1917). Introductory lectures on psycho-analysis (Part III). In J. Strachey (Ed.), *The Standard Edition of the Complete Psychological Works of Sigmund Freud, Volume XVI (1916–1917)*. London, England: Hogarth Press.

Lacan, J. (2006a). The direction of the treatment and the principle of its power. In *Écrits* (pp. 489–542). New York: W.W. Norton and Company.

Lacan, J. (2006b). The function and field of speech and language in psychoanalysis. In *Écrits* (pp. 197–268). New York: W.W. Norton and Company.

Lacan, J. (2006c). On a question prior to any possible treatment of psychosis. In *Écrits* (pp. 445–488). New York: W.W. Norton and Company.

Lacan, J. (2017). *Formations of the Unconscious. The Seminar of Jacques Lacan, Book V*. Cambridge, UK: Polity Press.

Meyer, C. (2011). Speech, language, and savoir in the Lacanian clinic of addiction. In *Lacan and Addiction: An Anthology*. London, Great Britain: Karnac.

Miller, J.A. (1991). The analytic experience: Means, ends, and results. In *Lacan and the Subject of Language* (pp. 83–99). New York: Routledge.

Chapter 6

The Enigmatic Body and the Constitution of Immigrants' Identity and Subjectivity

Debora Kirschbaum Nitkin

Introduction

Immigration may drastically disrupt and complexify one's experiences of the body. It exemplarily illustrates the intrinsic disjunction between being and body, which may be obscured in Cartesian approaches, such as the current medical discourse and its emphasis on the biological body (Clavreul 1983; Miller 2019). This happens because immigrating involves shifts in lifestyle, cultural references and values, language use, allocation in the labour market, and interpersonal relationships that affect significantly one's subjectivity and identity (Hamad and Melman 2019). Sometimes, these changes are experienced at the level of the body through the formation of bodily manifestations. For example, research shows that Canadian immigrants' physical and mental health tends to decline after the first five years since their arrival to Canada, a phenomenon called "Healthy Immigrant Effect" (Lu and Ng 2019).

I observe resonances of this phenomenon in my clinical work with new or established immigrants, who often complain about bodily manifestations, such as gastrointestinal issues, headaches, leg pain, or skin and panic attacks, whose onset they associate with the post-immigration event. Strikingly, many of these cases were first diagnosed as "unexplained medical symptoms" (Kyrmayer et al. 2004:663), after medical tests excluded the presence of anatomic or physiological alteration. This finding overwhelms those individuals, baffling them with a strong sense of disbelief and mystifying them with a worry at not understanding the medical results. Combined, these feelings propel the newcomer to seek psychotherapy in search of a response to the "reality" of those body manifestations.

Would those puzzlements and disbelief be influenced or worsened by the loss of cultural references that might equip these persons to make meaning of body manifestations in the new social context? Would they be expressions of the person's lack of resources for putting words to the experience of encountering a new sociocultural context, a new Other?[1] How would be possible to understand those enigmatic experiences from a psychoanalytical viewpoint?

DOI: 10.4324/9781003212072-7

Turning our lens to the constitution of identity and subjectivity may provide a deeper and unique insight into the complexity that involves the experience of the body.

The focus of this chapter is the conceptualization of the body and its articulation through body manifestations that concern the field of subjectivity and identity as articulated by Jacques Lacan (1991, 2014), in order to elucidate how they might be impacted by immigration, as an encounter with the Other (Hamad and Melman 2019).

I argue that that incredulity and momentary suspension of meaning making about those body manifestations may be expressions of struggles in the encounter with a new outside world and attempts at establishing social bonds with it.

Immigration and Body Experience

The notion of body is central in the psychoanalytical conceptualization of the human experience (Miller 2016, 2019) as it plays a pivotal role in the constitution of identity and subjectivity, two dimensions that are more directly affected in the experience of immigration. When a person moves from her home country and loses her mother tongue, social network, professional career, cultural references, and so on, the body is the only thing other than personal belongings that she keeps with her (Hamad and Melman 2019; Kyrmayer et al. 2009). Such experience illuminates Lacan's (2018) argument that we have a body, rather than that we are a body.

"To have a relationship with one's own body as though it were foreign is certainly a possibility, one that is expressed by the use of the verb *to have*. One has one's body." (Lacan 2018:129)

Because of the displacement of cultural and linguistic references it provokes (Hamad and Melman 2019), immigration disrupts the egoic alienation in which one lives, as the person engages in a process of redefining her identity, seen, until then, as a given. For example, one's name may be written or pronounced differently from what one was used to (Hamad and Melman 2019). One's outlook and personality traits – which served to distinguish one from everyone else in one's social network in the home country – are no longer known for the new peers. A person instead starts to be designated by major social categories (Vanheule and Verhaehghe 2009), such as nationality, gender, race, career, degrees, and so on, to which one may not see oneself as completely belonging. Or, further, a person's style or appearance may change due to engagement in new eating habits, dress codes, social conventions, etc. Over time, a person may feel strange or uncomfortable in her own skin; for example, after experiencing significant change in body shape due to weight gain and sedentariness during winter, distraught immigrants have told me: "This is not me". These kinds of remarks, which I notice in clinical practice, are corroborated by evidence-based research.

Life changes faced after immigrating to Canada significantly impact immigrants' physical and mental health (Kyrmayer et al. 2009). Research on the Healthy Immigrant Effect has shown how significantly immigrants' health conditions decline over time after moving to Canada, in spite of being healthier than the general Canadian-born population at the time of their arrival, as assessed through medical screening tests prior to their admission (Kyrmayer et al. 2009). These studies speculate that the worsening of immigrants' health conditions, detected through the HIE, may be attributed to "difficulties in adjusting to new environment, stress and/or adoption of risky health behaviours" (Lu and Ng 2019).

Many of the studies on the health of immigrants in Canada show that struggles to adjust to a new environment may comprise myriad issues that range from challenges in adjusting to new climate conditions, to problems with communicating due to language barriers, difficulties in navigating the cultures of new workplaces and/or educational institutions, obtaining professional licencing credentials, and so on (Kyrmayer et al. 2009). They also depict significant lifestyle changes in terms of eating habits, physical activities, leisure, social interactions, and cultural and religious values that may contribute to the deterioration of health conditions of recent or established immigrants in Canada (Kyrmayer et al. 2009; Lu and Ng 2019). In addition to these issues, social isolation, lack of a social support network, difficulties in finding employment or being unable to work in the profession(s) practiced in the native country, racism, and lack of access to timely primary health care are some of the factors that may contribute to increasing levels of stress and the aforementioned "risky health behaviours" (Lu and Ng 2019). Among the health issues that most affect immigrants' mental health, researchers point out depression, anxiety, post-traumatic stress disorder, and medically unexplained symptoms, "particularly pain, fatigue, and gastrointestinal and genitourinary symptoms" (Kyrmayer et al. 2009).

The question remaining is how the emergence of these body manifestations intersects with "adjustments" needed at the level of subjectivity and identification that immigrants must make in order "to fit in" with the host society, which may go beyond the concept of identity (Vanheule and Verhaehghe 2009:392). According to Vanheule and Verhaehghe (2009), the inherent problem created by this concept is that one uses it to mean "collective belonging" (p. 393), and in doing so we tend to refer to a norm to which anyone should adhere in order to belong. This norm casts one's subjectivity as a frame that defines what one is, based on comparisons between different people. Categories such as gender, ethnicity, race, and social class produce this type of effect in the construction of identity as such; this blurs the nuances that mark each individual's trajectory, that is, what is singular to each person, such as one's body experience. In order to understand in-depth this intricate process, we will delve into the conceptualization of identification, subjectivity, and the body and their intrinsic interrelationship from a psychoanalytical perspective.

The Body Experience From a Psychoanalytical Perspective

The Body as Image

Freud's initial clinical work on neuroses and psychoneurosis led him to the recognition that the I, or Ego,[2] was a formation involving complex processes produced throughout the early phases of one's psychosexual development. He coined narcissism, the phase in which the function of the I is configured as an autonomous entity; subsequently, the previous stage of auto-eroticism (Freud 1957b). Lacan (2006a) built on but innovated Freud's insight by arguing that the formation of the I not only succeeded the constitution of a body image but also consisted of a logical operation.

Lacan coined "the mirror stage" (2006a:94) to describe that logical operation, incorporating the advancements of 1930s neurobiology in its formulation. The stage corresponds to a temporal moment in which the infant, held by the mother (or her substitute) in front of a mirror, eventually recognizes that the reflected image is, indeed, her own, rather than another baby, as the child previously and erroneously thought. This moment is also marked by the presence of the mother's gaze and voice, towards which the infant turns in search of confirmation of the child's deduction that the image belongs to him or her. The mother's gaze validates the child's inference, and it is also internalized as something concerning to his or her body. This inaugurates the child's entrance in both imaginary and symbolic order; this happens to children around ages 6–18 months (Lacan 2006a).

This operation is foundational for providing a unity to the body that, until then, was experienced as fragmented. According to Lacan (2006a), this fragmentation results from both the child's neurological immaturity and the libidinization of the child's body through the provision of maternal care. Neurological immaturity would impede visualization of the object reflected in the mirror in its entirety in the earlier stage, and the libidinization, still in progress, imprints traces only on parts of the body, which hinders the imaginarization (Dunker 2018) of the body as unity until the conclusion of the mirror stage.

The implications of this operation for the constitution of one's identity, subjectivity, and experience of body are key because it shows that all go beyond the limits of the psychological realm and the biological organism, as it is articulated within the realm of science (Lacan 1998a). Lacan argues that the body is, above all, an image, whose configuration relies on libidinal investments resulting from maternal care. This is why one's experience of identity is an experience of alienation inasmuch as one is able to recognize oneself only as an image of an "other" (Lacan 1991). However, its existence as "I" also relies on recognition from an Other, then represented by the mother. Years later, he synthesized the novelty of his contribution as follows:

> whatever in man is loosened up, fragmented, anarchic, establishes its relation to his perception on a plane with a completely original tension. The image of his body is the principle of every unity he perceives in objects. Now, he only perceives the unity of this specific image from the outside, and in anticipated manner. Because of this double relation which he has with himself, all the objects of his world are always structured around the wandering shadow of his own ego. . . . Man's ideal unity, which is never attained as such and escapes him at every moment, is evoked . . . in this perception.
>
> (Lacan 1991:166)

This man's position triggers the onset of consecutive identifications that will progressively make up one's identity.

Identification and Body Experience

Identification is a notion originally created by Freud (1957a) to describe a process in which one unconsciously resembles totally or partially aspects of another person's outlook, behaviour, or symptomatic manifestations (Chemama 1997). This conceptualization was later rearticulated by Freud (Chemama 1997) to describe how someone incorporates certain elements in particular that were peculiar to another person who was either loved, or detested, or indifferent to the production of a symptomatic manifestation. This notion was crucial for explaining the formation of body manifestations, such as aphonia, paralysis, and fainting, presented by Freud's first cases of hysteria (1957a). Those symptoms were initially unexplained from a medical viewpoint due to the lack of any physical cause. However, Freud realized that, curiously, some of those patients' significant others had previously presented those symptoms. This led him to hypothesize that the patients unconsciously enacted those symptoms to bring to his attention an issue that concerned their relationship to those significant others, yet in a camouflaged way. Freud (1957a) concluded that the hysterics were identified with another person who either possessed a position in which they wished to be, or not to be, and that they have refrained from pursuing due to thinking that it was morally unacceptable. Therefore, the symptom was an indirect and intricate way of communicating unpleasant ideas that referred to those whose behaviours might have caused their suffering and anxiety. They tended to disappear as soon as the patient spoke about the conflict in response to Freud's interpretations. Subsequently, Freud realized that the process of identification was not limited to hysteria but was also present in other neurosis, as well as being a constituent element of psychosexual development (Freud1957b)

Lacan refined Freud's theorization on identification in order to advance the understanding of the formation of the I. For Lacan (2014), identification operates in two dimensions: one in the imaginary, the other in the symbolic order. The "imaginary identification" (Lacan 2014:37) is the one in which the child recognizes herself in the stage of the mirror, and that operation forms the basis for the constitution of an ego-ideal, as well as the one observed in the hysteric's identification. "Symbolic identification" (Lacan 2015:355) is the one referred to as a "single trait"[3] (Lacan 2015:352), the "*einziger Zug*", in German. This is a sign that reflects what is radically different in this subject from all the others existing in a set and that makes this person absolutely singular. Lacan explains that this single trait is a sign and not a signifier because it cannot be linked back, afterwards, to another signifier, generating a "signifying battery" (2015:355), or evoking other ones. According to Lacan, "what is defined by this *ein einziger Zug* is the punctual character of the early reference to the Other when it comes to narcissism" (Lacan 2015:355). Lacan's hypothesis, at that time, was that it would be the internalization of the gaze of the Other by the child, in the very moment the child makes the choice between the child in the Other's arms and its specular image, that constitutes the single trait, that is, the subject's pure difference (Lacan 2015).

After this, almost everything concerned the ego-ideal, the utmost development of the specular image; the ideal-ego is related to the identifications that one engages in throughout one's life. For Lacan (2015), the ego-ideal is the result of an imaginary projection, while the ideal-ego, or ideal I, is a symbolic introjection. The narcissistic satisfaction that unfolds in the relationship between the ego and the ego-ideal relies always on the possibility of referring to the ideal-ego (Lacan 2015:356), which represents cultural norms, the father's law, and social approval. However, in the 1960s, Lacan would refine these ideas and contend that the base of symbolic identification is identification with the object of desire, which he designates as *a* (Lacan 2014:37). This a, written in lower case, initially was a reference to the small other, "autre" in French, that designates the ego and, eventually, was used to refer to the *objet petit a*, as the object cause of desire (Lacan 2014).

The Spoken Body

In the 1950s, Lacan (2006b) conceives the body as a body spoken by the Other of the language. As language precedes one's existence, the child is spoken of in the languages in which parents and their predecessors talk and dream about a soon-to-be child. Therefore, before being born, one already occupies a place in the Other, inscribed in the Other's desire.

This inclusion corresponds to an affiliation, a membership, that anchors the subject and provides recognition to it in the field of the Other, which makes symbolic identifications possible. For example, the name that one receives at one's birth, the "proper name", plays a key role in the constitution of the first signifier, S1, as it is invested by significations projected by the parents. The proper name is equated by Lacan (1991) to the unary trait in the symbolic identification, and it is central in the constitution of the subject.

The conceptualization of the subject and the Other as language marked another turning point in Lacan's teaching. Lacan (1991) shifted the focus from the intersubjective relationship to the unconscious and its structure as a language (Lacan 2005b). He argued that the emphasis on the imaginary contributed to distancing psychoanalysts from the alma mater of its work with unconscious formations, which was key to grasp the clinical phenomena. Lacan (2006b) contended that a return to Freud's earlier studies about the unconscious was imperative to substantiate more robustly his initial insights about the symbolic order. Freud used the term unconscious to refer to the instance of the mind where the representatives of repressed thoughts about sexuality were stored in the psychic apparatus (Lacan 2006b; Chemama 1997). In the beginning of his work, he realized that neurotic symptoms resembled the organization of dreams, jokes, and rebuses, in which ideas corresponding to sexual desire and affects, considered morally unacceptable for the individual, would be distorted, inverted, and camouflaged by the speaker in way that would hinder recognition of the original thought. For Lacan (2006b, 2006c), Freud realized that those changes followed a rationality and patterns, and named these different operations repression, condensation, and displacement.

Lacan (2006b) built on these ideas to demonstrate that the unconscious phenomena at stake in the relationship of analyst–analysand, and in the symptom, were an effect of the structure of the language; this was what allowed the former to unpack the latter. The language is incarnated in speech, the unfolding of a signifying chain, which had to be listened to closely to capture the meaning of one's unconscious desire, rather finding it in the depths of a metaphysical psychic apparatus. Lacan (2006b) argued that the symptom should be approached as a linguistic sign, as conceptualized by Ferdinand Saussure, but proposed that the signifier should have primacy over the signified. He posited that the signified might correspond to several diverse and unanticipated meanings, opposing Saussure's thesis regarding a univocal relation between signified and signifier. Those insights allowed Lacan (2006b) to assert that the formation of the psychoanalytical symptoms resembled the mechanisms observed in figures of language, such as metaphor and metonymy, and allowed him to replace Freud's notions of condensation and displacement.

These developments represented a turning point in the theory for the conceptualization of the body as the prominence of the image was substituted by the determination of the signifier. He equated the body to the language:

> Speech is in fact a gift of language, and language is not immaterial. It is a subtle body, but body it is. Words are caught up in all the body images that captivate the subject; they may knock up the hysteric, be identified with the object of Penisneid, . . . , or represent the feces retained in avaricious *jouissance*. Furthermore, words themselves can suffer symbolic lesions and accomplish imaginary acts whose victim is the subject.
>
> (Lacan 2006b:248)

That "subtle body" was observed in the "somatic compliance" (Freud 1957a:105) featured in the conversion symptoms of the hysteria, for example, and the materiality of the signifier was crucial to account for the formation of the hysteric body, which was a body shaped by language Zucchi (2015), a fictional body. The materiality of the signifier was also revealed in the somatizations presented by Freud's obsessional patients, such as the Wolf Man and the Rat Man (Lacan 2006b). For Lacan, this indicated that the symptom, shaped as a ciphered message, had the function of communicating the unconscious desire subjacent to it. As Lacan (2006b: 232) explains:

> Hieroglyphics of hysteria, blazons of phobia and labyrinths of Zwangsneurose [obsessive neurosis]; charms of impotence, enigmas of inhibition, and oracles of anxiety; talking arms of character, seals of punishment and disguises of perversion: these are elements that our exegesis resolves, . . .

Closely listening to the speech would provide access to that message. Nevertheless, the materiality of the signifier was not sufficient for eliminating the evanescence that characterizes the subject of the unconscious, and Lacan suggested that the letter was the body of the significant and, therefore, the signifying chain that corresponded to a spoken body (Lacan 2006c).

Reframing Freud's notion of desire in light of Hegel's conceptualization of desire as "desire for the desire of the Other", Lacan (2006d:689, 2014) stated that the subject is the place in which the desire manifests itself as a lack: a lack that marks the place where something that concerns both the desire of the Other and the one designated by the single trait (S1). The concept "subject" refers to an effect of language (Lacan 2006d) in which a void emerges in the signifying chain that constitutes one's speech. The subject is what occupies it, and the signifier represents the subject for another signifier (Lacan 2006d). So, one can only speak about one's desire by referring to the Other's desire for desire. The Other, then, represents the "treasure of signifiers" (Lacan 2006d) available in the language, which includes both the mother tongue and the foreign languages spoken in that cultural context.

The problem contained in the dialectic of desire is that the subject can only know about its desire by questioning what the Other's desire is – *Che vuoi?* (Lacan 2006d:390). E.g., a child can only determine the child's desire out by asking what the mother wants, and then trying to shape herself according to what she supposes will satisfy that desire. However, the child articulates her demand by using the signifiers provided by the child's mother and others to whom the child is exposed in the process of socialization and acquisition of the language. This limitation catapults the subject in an intrinsic condition of alienation as its desire cannot be articulated, unless when referring to the desire of someone else. The subject seeks to escape from this impasse by searching for the lack in the Other and offering itself to fill it in, but it is unsuccessful because what the Other desires is a lack. This lack arises from the impossibility of representing the completeness in the Other, which is the result of the incidence of the sexual division in which there is either the possession of the phallus or its absence. The question about whether or not one is this object, or has this object that might veil the lack in the Other, is the issue subjacent to that dialectic. This creates an impasse as one eventually realizes that that desire is still not one's own. Consequently, the unsubstantiality found at the level of the ego is reencountered here in the level of the subject, and he asserts that the human condition is permanently a position of lack, to which man responds by either seeking to veil his own lack in the body or veiling the lack in the Other.

Body as Jouissance

In the 1960s, Lacan (1998, 2014) again changed his theorization about the unconscious and the notion of body. He observed that the never-ending possibility of signifying the encounter with the "rock of castration" – a symbolic operation that marks the resolution of the Oedipal phase and the subject's realization that the sexual difference overdetermines one's impossibility of completeness, and the reality of the division of the subject – due to the structure of the language created difficulties for the termination of the analysis. Lacan turned his efforts to the investigation of the element that was unrepresentable, but never stopped to return to the formation of the symptoms. Lacan hypothesized that this element was the ultimate cause of the desire and coined it "object a" (*objet petit a*) (Lacan 2014:40). He showed how it plays an important function in the formation of anxiety and how it takes over one's body, producing diverse body manifestations, such as the ones observed in panic attacks. The object *a* has to do with a part of the body that in the mirror stage remains excluded from the image of the I, that is, a leftover from the imagination of the real body. Lacan (2014:40) states that:

> I manipulated this surface in front of you . . . to form an idea of how the cut can establish two different pieces here, one which can have a specular image and the other which quite literally, doesn't have one. It was a question of the relationship between minus-*phi* and the constitution of the little *a*. On one hand, there is the reserve that can't be grasped in the imaginary, even though it is linked to an organ, . . . , this instrument which will all the same to go into action . . . for the satisfaction of desire, the phallus. On the other hand, there is the a, which is this remainder, this residue, this object whose status escapes the status of the object derived from the specular image. . . . This object a whose constituent characteristics we have merely touched on . . . is what is in question whenever Freud speaks about the object in connection with anxiety.

Lacan's formulation of what was at stake in the formation of anxiety, in the light of Shakespeare's *Hamlet*, led him to conclude that the cause of the former was not a lack of object, as previously thought by Freud, but, indeed, the presence of the object that represents the lack, that is, the object *a*. Lacan (1998a) refined this conceptualization during *Seminar* XI, in which he articulated the nature of the object a in light of Velazques' painting, "Las Meninas". In this artwork, we can observe the painter painting the models through an open door and the studio where this scene is played. Lacan (1998a) argues that the object *a* is that place occupied by the gaze of the spectator and transposes this example to the explanation of what is at stake in the formation of one's body experience, as the gaze of the Other, or the gaze of the mother in the case of the stage of the mirror, is captured by the subject as part of the body image. However, this place marks the absence of the object, as where there was the eye, there is a gaze instead. The enjoyment that being gazed by this Other produces in the moment that one recognizes the reflected image as being one's own is the experience that one tries to repeat endlessly throughout one's life. This leads to Lacan's new articulation of the body experience as the experience of being body subjected to the gaze, and also a body that is invested by "*jouissance*" (Lacan 1998a) – a French word that describes a kind of enjoyment, for which there is not a corresponding word in English. The object a, then, becomes as the phallus, the place in the Other where there is a lack, which the subject attempts to fill in by offering itself as the object that completes what is missing in the Other, although unsuccessfully.

Body as Speaking Body

In the 1970s, Lacan (2018) argued that the term "unconscious" was misleading for describing this instance of the mind where the representation of the being's incompleteness dwells and suggested substitution for the notion "speaking body". After his death, Lacanian psychoanalysts led by Miller (2016, 2019) have thrived on elucidating this idea. They contend that the contemporary fall of the patriarchal order and its ideals, observed since the late 20th century, has catapulted us into a post-Oedipal era, in which the reference to universal norms and truth has been replaced by plural and diversified ways of living. Consequently, there is a weakness of the Other, and its replacement for multiple different ones. The individuals are each time less inclined to seek signification, and more compelled to engage in body manifestations, which cannot be interpreted in the same way as in the 20th century, as they are not organized based on universal norms. Miller (2016) called these body manifestations "new symptoms". Their main feature is the subject's engagement in modes of enjoyment that involve excess, and they are experienced strictly in the level of the body with very limited or no connection to meaning. This is why Miller (2019, 2016) states that these symptoms have an incidence on the real of the body. Addictions, panic attacks, bulimia, anorexia, and other psychosomatic phenomena exemplify those new symptoms, which might be understood as attempts at articulating the castration anxiety that results from the dissolution of the borders that earlier on were sustained by the Name-of-the-Father. One of the problems introduced by the new symptoms is that the psychoanalytical intervention must transcend the ambit of the Symbolic register and operate at the level of the Real (Miller 2016). As the Real is the realm where the representations are absent, the new symptoms are shaped by the erratic circulation of partial drives around the *objet petit a* that makes up the *jouissance*. As a result, the interpretations consist more of interventions that target the body than interpretations that aim at meaning, and so must be done on a case-by-case basis (Miller 2016). The objective is to reduce the experience of the subject to what is unique about that subject, making its way of enjoying distinguishable from everyone else. The subject is encouraged to take responsibility for its choices concerning its *jouissance*, which are not connected to meaning and purpose but rather to being content about being. This is what gives some consistency to the speaking body that supports the *parlêtre* (Lacan 2018; Miller 2016), that is, the speaking being, and is the contemporary shape taken by the unconscious.

The Intricacies of Having a Body

The previous discussion about the complexity that involves the body experience provides the elements to discuss in greater depth the phenomena involving the emergence of body manifestations experienced by immigrants.

Vignette

M.B.P.X. moved from South America to Canada with her partner and children, seeking quality of life. In her home country, she had an excellent job in finance and was renowned for being a competent, professional, and warm woman. Her degree in accounting, in addition to her proficiency in English, made her a successful applicant for Permanent Residency (PR) in Canada. Months later, she was hired by a financial institution, and one year after that, to her surprise, she was invited to accept an executive position. She decided to abbreviate her name to make it easier to sign documents. Her family responsibilities and heavy workload led her to abandon her previous healthy lifestyle. She and her partner stopped cooking at home and started to consume processed food, as it was time saving. She neglected exercising in order to work more hours and achieve more recognition in her work. M.B.P.X. started the process of obtaining Canadian credentials, which she believed would allow her to remain in the executive position. One day, she felt a pressure in her chest and palpitations, and had cold sweats in the middle of a presentation. These symptoms reappeared twice during that week. Scared, she thought that they could be the result of stress and went to the Emergency Department. All medical tests came back negative. She continued to experience these symptoms. She returned to the emergency and went to her family doctor, but again, there was no medical explanation found. She was encouraged to take anxiolytic medication and look for therapy. It took her a long time to seek it out, and she was very reluctant to initiate psychological treatment because she was convinced that the doctors had missed something. She started therapy and complained about the difficulties that this situation created for her interpersonal relationships and public speaking. She became withdrawn and short tempered. New symptoms appeared. She suffered from gastrointestinal problems and had difficulty swallowing. For a long period, she struggled to make sense of the psychoanalyst's interpretations, and in response to them, the panic attacks became more frequent. As time went by, she gained more insight into the power dynamics in the host society and started to establish links between the physical symptoms and her feelings of alienation. She realized that she could not swallow the new lifestyle that she had imposed on herself.

This vignette portrays some of the challenges that the subject faces in the encounter with the new Other and the disruption that it brings at the level of the Imaginary, Symbolic, and Real registers, highlighting issues concerning identification, desire, and *jouissance* that contribute to the emergence of the body manifestations. M.B.P.X.'s initial struggles with finding meaning suggested that those panic attacks and somatizations were a manifestation of new symptoms and ways of expressing her *jouissance* for disappearing as an accomplished speaker on those occasions when she had to speak. However, over the course of the treatment, it became clearer that those body manifestations might have been seen as classical symptoms of anxiety and conversion disorder if M.P.B.X.'s system of cultural references was not so destabilized due to her lack of knowledge about the social arrangement that supported the power dynamics in which she was involved. Her conditions of interpreting the Other's desire, which is always impossible, were shut down as she attempted to articulate her demand based on imaginary identifications. For example, she burned out working long hours, seeking credentials that, supposedly, would make her more desirable for the Other, incarnated in the financial institution, professional boards, and the host country's social order, as she imagined that this was what people in her new social network expected from her. In order to look like everybody else in her work environment and community, she changed her name, adopting an abbreviation that made hard for her to recognize herself when she was referred to by others. She changed her lifestyle to match Others' ways of functioning, as she imagined that by becoming "more efficient", her chances of filling the lack in the Other would increase.

The body manifestations that she started to suffer from were ways of expressing her desire to fulfil the desire of the Other and to avoid her anxiety over feeling unable to do so due to her recognition of incompleteness.

Conclusion

The complexity of the body experience becomes evident when we seek to grasp it in light of the phenomena implicated in immigration. Body manifestations that emerge during this process show that the body is experienced by human beings in ways that go beyond the biological organism of the medical discourse. The consistency of the body as a theoretical category that is foundational in the human experience as an identarian and subjective phenomenon is formalized within the developments of the psychoanalytical discourse originally formulated by Jacques Lacan. Approaching the body from such a perspective opens up the possibility of recognizing that our identity and subjective experiences are intrinsically intertwined with the body in its Imaginary, Symbolic, and Real dimensions. This understanding permits us to deepen our understanding that certain body manifestations imply attempts to reallocate ourselves within a still unknown social order, and that, when unheard, hinder one's capacity to establish social bonds with the Other, whose desire remains enigmatic. From a Lacanian perspective, those body expressions sometimes correspond to a repackaging of classical body manifestations, which may resemble earlier processes of constitution of the subject, and aim to give consistency to one's body. They emerge as new forms of building links with an Other that does not sustain universal ideals anymore, and because of this opens up the possibility of reinventing oneself and taking responsibility for one's unique way of enjoying the body as real.

Notes

1 The "Other" is a conceptual category that accounts for what is outside the subject, that is, language, social order, and "unconscious".
2 The instance of our psychical life that corresponds to our identity as human beings.
3 The terms unary trait and single trait are used interchangeably by English translators.

Works Cited

Chaohui, Lu and Edward Ng. 2019. "Healthy Immigrant Effect by Immigrant Category in Canada". *Health Reports. Statistics Canada*, Catalogue No. 82-003-X. Retrieved December 17, 2019 (https://www150.statcan.gc.ca/n1/en/pub/82-003-x/2019004/article/00001-eng.pdf?st=KpAP_2Uf.pdf).

Chemama, Roland. 1997. *Dictionnaire de la Psychanalyse*. Paris: Larousse.

Clavreul, Jean. 1983. *A Ordem Médica: Poder e impotência do discurso médico*. Translated by J. Noujain, M.A.C. Jorge and P.M. Silveira. Sao Paulo: Braziliense.

Dunker, Christian. 2018. *The Constitution of the Psychoanalytic Clinic: A History of Its Structure and Power*. Retrieved October 2019 (www.taylorfrancis.com/books/9780429481352.)

Freud, Sigmund. 1957a. "Fragment of an Analysis of a Case of Hysteria". Pp. 3–124 in *The Standard Edition of the Complete Psychological Works of Sigmund Freud*, Vol. VII (1901–1905), A Case of Hysteria, Three Essays on Sexuality and Other Works, edited and translated by J. Strachey and A. Freud, 3–124. London: Hogarth Press and the Institute of Psychoanalysis.

Freud, Sigmund. 1957b. "On Narcissism: An Introduction". Pp. 67–102 in *The Standard Edition of the Complete Psychological Works of Sigmund Freud*, Vol. XIV (1914–1916), On the History of the Psycho-analytic Movement, Papers on Metapsychology and Other Works, edited and translated by J. Strachey and A. Freud, 67–102. London: Hogarth Press and the Institute of Psychoanalysis.

Hamad, Nazir and Charles Melman. 2019. *Psicologia da Imigração*. Sao Paulo: Instituto Langage.

Kyrmayer, Laurence, Danielle Groleau, Karl Looper and Melissa D. Dao. 2004. "Explaining Medically Unexplained Symptoms". *Canadian Journal of Psychiatry*, 49 (10): 663–672.

Kyrmayer, L., L. Narasiah, M. Munoz, M. Rashid, M.A. Ryder and K. Pottie. 2009. "Common Mental Health Problems in Immigrants and Refugees: General Approach in Primary Care". *Canadian Medical Association Journal*, 183 (12): 959–967. doi:10.1503/cmaj.090292

Lacan, Jacques. 1991. *The Seminar of Jacques Lacan, Book II. The Ego in Freud's Theory and in the Technique of Psychoanalysis, 1954–1955*. Edited by J.A. Miller and translated by S. Tomaselli. New York: W.W. Norton.

Lacan, Jacques. 1998a. *The Seminar of Jacques Lacan, book XI. The Four Fundamental Concepts of Psychoanalysis, 1964*. Edited by and Jacques Alain Miller and translated by Alan Sheridan. New York: W.W. Norton.

Lacan, Jacques. 1998b. *The Seminar of Jacques Lacan, Book XX. The Feminine Sexuality. The Limits of Love and Knowledge, 1972–1973*. Edited by and Jacques Alain Miller and translated by Alan Sheridan. New York: W.W. Norton.

Lacan, Jacques. 2006a. *The Mirror Stage as Formative of the I Function as Revealed in Psychoanalytic Experience*. In *Écrits*, Translated by B. Fink. New York: W.W. Norton.

Lacan, Jacques. 2006b. *The Function and Field of Speech and Language in Psychoanalysis*. In *Écrits*, Translated by B. Fink. New York: W.W. Norton.
Lacan, Jacques. 2006c. *The Instance of the Letter in the Unconscious*. In *Écrits*, Translated by B. Fink. New York: W.W. Norton.
Lacan, Jacques. 2006d. *The Subversion of the Subject and the Dialectic of Desire*. In *Écrits*, Translated by B. Fink. New York: W.W. Norton.
Lacan, Jacques. 2014. *The Seminar of Jacques Lacan, Book X. Anxiety, 1962–1963*. Edited by J.A. Miller and translated by A.R. Price. Cambridge, Malden: Polity Press.
Lacan, Jacques. 2015. *The Seminar of Jacques Lacan, Book VIII. Transference, 1960–1961*. Edited by J.A. Miller and translated by B. Fink. Cambridge, Malden: Polity Press.
Lacan, Jacques. 2018. *The Seminar of Jacques Lacan, Book XXIII. The Sinthome, 1975–1976*. Edited by J.A. Miller and translated by A.R.Price. Cambridge, Malden: Polity Press.
Lu, Chaohui and Edward Ng. 2019. "Healthy Immigrant Effect by Immigrant Category in Canada". *Health Reports*, 30 (4): 3–11. https://doi.org/10.25318/82-003-x201900400001-eng
Miller, Jacques-Alain. 2016. *The Unconscious and the Speaking Body*. Retrieved August 2019 (www.wapol.org/en/articulos/Template.asp?intTipoPagina=4&intPublicacion=13&intEdicion=9&intIdiomaPublicacion=2&intArticulo=2742&intIdiomaArticulo=2).
Miller, Jacques-Alain. 2019. *Lacanian Biology and the Event of the Body*. Part I. The Symptom. 18. Retrieved September 2019 (www.lacan.com/symptom/lacanian-biology-miller/).
Vanheule, Stijn and Verhaehghe Paul. 2009. "Identity Through a Psychoanalytic Looking Glass". *Theory and Psychology*, 19 (3): 391–411.
Zucchi, Marcia. 2015. *Outro Corpo: Inconsciente, Sintoma e a Clínica do Corpo*. Rio de Janeiro: KBR. Retrieved January 2020 (www.amazon.ca/Outro-corpo-Inconsciente-Sintoma-Portuguese-ebook/dp/B0171049RQ-Ebook).

Chapter 7

A Conversation on Psychoanalytic Work with Children in the System[1]

Kristen Hennessy and Chris Vanderwees

Chris Vanderwees (CV): How would you describe the Lacanian approach and what it brings to your clinical practice with children and adolescents?

Kristen Hennessy (KH): I think that what it brings is respect for the subject. Kids do not bring themselves for treatment. There is always someone else saying, "this is a child who needs treatment." I think many other approaches, even psychoanalytic approaches, see the child's symptom as something to be removed. A Lacanian approach does a better job in treating the child with respect and seeing the child as a person in his or her own right as opposed to an object that belongs to the parent. There are many ways that this can be done in a technical sense, but it is also about an attitude towards treatment and how the treatment functions. It is little things like asking even a 3-year-old at the end of the consultation, "would you like to return?" It could also be about not agreeing with the adults as to the goals of treatment for the child.

CV: When you say the respect for the subject, is there an implication that often we do not listen to children? Do you encounter this often in your work, that is, people not listening to what the child has to say?

KH: I think we often do not listen to children and we should. The children with whom I work are in foster care, so I am interacting with their biological parents and foster parents. There is a wide range. Some parents have no interest in listening to children. There are others who are wonderful at listening to children and who are interested and able to engage with me in a way that is wondering about the child as opposed to changing the child. There are also people who want to listen but struggle to do it, and would need their own analysis in order to be able to hear. Of course, we have the old expression, "children are to be seen and not heard." Although this is a more old-fashioned idea about child rearing, I do think a lot of parents I work with grew up with this sort of attitude, which has now made it difficult for them to listen to children.

The system also often does not listen to children. There is one county, for instance, where all children are required to attend court hearings – even toddlers. When foster parents complain, the county will say, "well,

DOI: 10.4324/9781003212072-8

the child does not know what is going on." I had one young patient erupt into a wail in the middle of a hearing and people said, "how did they know the child was crying because of the hearing?" Parents may struggle to listen to children, but the system also sometimes forgets that children are subjects. This points to something else – families and systems often have the wish that the child's symptom is meaningless, and that it does not implicate anyone.

CV: There's not much hearing necessarily happening in the hearing.

KH: Right – and sometimes I will end up saying during a hearing, "my patient is a kid." This is something I say a lot: "my patient is a kid."

CV: Is this statement a response to an assumption occurring in the courtroom?

KH: It depends, but it seems that sometimes the fact that we are talking about the life of a child gets forgotten. It can devolve into conversations about rules and legal technicalities. The fact that the hearing is to discuss the life of a child can be forgotten pretty easily.

CV: How do you think about this notion of the mirror stage in your work? Is this concept of particular importance for you when working with children?

KH: I think about it especially in terms of the young children in foster care. In this context, there are two mirrors. There is the mirror of the biological family, which says, "this is who you are and this is who we want you to be." The child forms identifications based on that mirror. The law or someone else then steps in to say, "this family system is not okay or something here is not okay and now you are in this system." The mirror in this new system, however, is completely different. How the child is praised, criticized, and told about who they are is now different; what earned praise now earns criticism. There is a collapsing of the mirror that can happen. A child is told "this is who you are" and then they are moved somewhere else where everything changes. This becomes more complicated, for instance, when a child has been through nine or ten different homes. Although we could say there is a radical difference between the mirroring that happened in the abusive home and in the foster home – further, some foster homes are also abusive – it is important to remember that each family has their own individual and unique set of values.

When we talk about the image, it can be startling. People change the way that children look. I'll have a patient who comes to me in long scraggly hair and sweatpants. This is the child's style until they move and come in with braided hair and skirts. These changes are very much on the child's body. Of course, there is also what the child does with these changes. Do they take it up when they move? Are they willing to change identifications every time they move to a new family? Is there an identification that they hold onto, which one is that, and why?

Perhaps no more than any other child, but the children who I work with are very reassured by mirroring phenomenon in sessions. I am thinking of a particular patient whose mirroring was confused as a result of one of the parents lying a lot about what was going on and would encourage the child to think and say that certain things were going on. This child has become confused about who they are. They have two different histories: the one that they know and the one they have been told. This kiddo is 4 and recently he started bringing his baby pictures to sessions. It is like he is going back. He brings these pictures and wants them to be admired. It seems as though he is looking for mirroring that untangles some of the other stuff that has happened. It is a tricky situation to be in. As a clinician, you don't want to be in the position of telling a kid who they are, but the role then becomes to say, "that's you" or some message to say, "that's you and you are acceptable," and to leave it for the child to fill in more. Let them filter the identifications that they have received elsewhere into something that works for them.

CV: With the notion of mirroring and listening to what you have said, I am also thinking about the idea of recognition or we might even speak about object constancy. A child leaves one family and may end up in a situation having to relearn how to gain recognition or be recognized all over again in a new way. How do you negotiate being in the role of providing or helping with this sort of recognition?

KH: Often I become the constant. One thing that is fortunate is that our child and youth services tend to be pretty good about keeping treatment consistent. I have heard from other clinicians that some patients will start with a new therapist every time they move with a new family. The child ends up having nine families, nine schools, and nine therapists. This does not happen here unless the child moves so far that it is impossible to continue, which is rare. I become the constant in the transference. They come here with all these other changes going on. They can choose whether or not to be the same here. This also becomes a place where their history of recognition is remembered – the previous versions of the child are known and talked about, allowing the child to be seen in a different way.

More than mirror phenomenon with these kids, I think about the father function. My youngest children are 3 years old. For a substantial portion of my caseload, questions of structure are very much open. Whatever the outcome is, 3-year-olds are not yet neurotic. There are 3-year-olds on the path to neurosis, moving along, but the things that happen for someone to choose neurosis have not yet happened at this young age. This means that the question of structure is alive and in process. Also, these are children who have been exposed to someone who has broken the law. This might be concrete and literal, but I am also saying that this is concrete and literal at a time when these processes lead to a child selecting their structure. I want to say it this way because I think it is important.

The phrase I have come to is that every child should be issued an invitation to neurosis. Neurosis should be something that is offered to the child. I think sometimes that this is part of my job, that is, to offer neurosis to a child whether or not they accept that invitation. For me, the process that seems to help get children there is about understanding something of the law. What I mean by this is that the law offers a set of limits on behaviour, but also protections. Both limits and protections are often very lacking for the children I work with. Their own behaviour feels pretty limitless and what has happened to them is beyond limits. It is kind of a might meets right situation for many of these children. The process or the offer, then, is that everyone gives that up. There are rules that apply to the child and apply to us.

CV: There is usually some idea in Lacanianism that structure is fixed. One cannot move between structures, for instance, from neurosis to psychosis. Is it possible to influence the development of psychical structure with young children?

KH: According to Lacanian theory, one cannot move structures as an adult, but nobody says that you are born with a structure. This would get into DSM-like ideas that would suggest that schizophrenia is biologically inherited. Moreover, no-one is born neurotic: neurosis is the result of a process. So, if we are not born with our structure, at what point does it become fixed?

CV: Perhaps this is the crucial question that you have just raised. The emphasis is not necessarily on some genetic inheritance, but rather that there is something to structure that might be socially or environmentally influenced at a very early age. Are there things that one could do to help a child along the way to having, as you say, an invitation to neurosis?

KH: I think this is the core of treatment for a lot of young children on the path to psychosis. I can describe what I mean by this. I'll start with a counterexample. One child comes to mind who is on a troubled path to neurosis. He saw his father as the name-of-the-father. His father, however, was subject to whim, which was not really a law, but the child experienced it as such. Even though the behaviour of the father was extraordinarily unpredictable, the child thought that there was a law that he wasn't understanding well enough and experienced guilt for the abuse he suffered. The child felt that he had broken the law and was being rightfully punished even though he could not figure out what the rules were supposed to be. Now, the child has to rework a lot about that, but there is already something about the law that is there.

In the case of another little guy who would be more at risk for psychosis, he sees it as an individual choice. Mommy is lawless. You can have sex with mommy. You can do whatever you want. You can run through the world naked, setting the world on fire, or you can live how the foster parents live. He does not see anything in the former as violating a law. It is like lawlessness reigns. He very much enjoys that. He has been hurt in that environment and many bad things happened, but the kid will say, "I like naked." For him, the word "naked" means all of that. It is not only about nudity, but also about lawlessness. Here, the process for the child becomes about surrendering some of those pleasures. There is some limiting of the child while also helping him to get a sense of all that can come from the fruits or benefits that one might have in neurosis. Children start to learn the pleasures of language and play. There is a grieving that can happen around this free libidinal limitlessness, but there is a whole new world that opens up to the child. Showing something of this new world is a lot of the work with tiny tots.

CV: When I think about psychoanalysis with children, the play is frequently talked about in the literature as parallel to free association. We are talking about play, but the Lacanian clinic is presumably a clinic of speech. What does the clinic become in play with children? What are your thoughts about this?

KH: Play is full of speech. Silent play happens, but it is pretty rare. Kids talk a lot while they play. All the layers are there. For example, a child with a significant person in her life named "Robert" might play about "robbering." There is cops and robbers play, playing about the law, but also this specific figure of Robert, and what robbing might mean specifically to this child. Sounds and phonemes become important. Another child, for instance, with a person in her life, "Pena," likes to play with a zebra. The zebra ends up having similar characteristics as Pena during playtime. It is important not to create such a distinction between play and language because there are both in the session with a child, if you are listening for it. Kids do free associate with their play and with their bodies. If you listen to the play the same way that you listen to speech, a lot of things can happen.

When working with teens or adults, if I don't know what to do yet or am not sure what is going on in the case, I can listen and listen and take my time. What I used to find difficult in working with children, for example, if you are a character in the game, you have to do something. I might whisper to a kid, "what did she say next?" Over time, you do learn enough of the language of the child's world. At a certain point, a child has told you so much of the speech of the parents that it is easier to use a linguistic intervention in the play. I'm less anxious than I used to be, but it is difficult at the beginning when playing with a puppet, for instance, to discern what that puppet's role ought to be in treatment.

CV: In his "Note on the Child," Lacan emphasizes the significance of the symptom in the family system. As you have said, many of the children who you are working with have perhaps been through several family systems. How do you make sense of this idea for clinical practice?

KH: When I am working with a kid who is about to be adopted after having been in one place for a long time, I am paying attention to shifts in the symptom. Sometimes the symptom changes and is addressed to new people. The symptom begins to address the adopted family more than the biological family. Sometimes there is a symptom that continues to address the biological family, solely. Understandably, people are always interested in attachment with kids in foster care and in the process of adoption. This is the question of who is the kid attached to and why, but I tend to think more in terms of a different question: to whom is the child's symptom speaking? This tells me a great deal about who matters to them. Which system is the child addressing here? Sometimes a child's symptom can evolve from one system to the next. The symptom may have addressed something in the biological family, but shifts to incorporate something of the adoptive family. Back to the mirror phenomenon, the child may be able to address both families with the symptom while not selecting either. It also shows a child's creativity to be able to morph a symptom. An 8-year-old might be tagging unconscious things in one family and tagging unconscious things in another family all at once. I think it points us to the brilliance of a child's unconscious.

CV: Attachment is a term that is used to describe all sorts of phenomena in the contemporary clinic. Frequently, attachment it is talked about as being the primary aspect of the treatment that is going to be helpful to the patient, that is, in terms of the therapeutic alliance or so-called relationship. How do you make sense of attachment theory in relation to your work?

KH: I think about how my patients are doing with the people raising them. Sometimes it might have to do with untangling identifications. If this person hurt you and had black hair and new mom has black hair . . . there are a lot of cases of mistaken identity that can happen with children who have been profoundly abused. There is a lot of working on this in sessions. Compared to attachment-focused therapists or other psychoanalytic traditions, I am not attending to this idea so much in sessions. I find that if I am respectful and focused on the child's communication, the relationship kind of rolls along. Obviously, there are bumps. Transference phenomena are popping up everywhere, but you can address those things and treatment rolls along. I want patients to trust and to be able to speak and play. I see my role as more facilitating a path for them to relate to other people.

One of my concerns with some attachment work is that the clinicians are doing very direct and involved things to help a child connect to a parent, which I understand. There are clinicians who say you are supposed to rock the child for 15 minutes, rub lotion on the child, and feed them a bottle. I don't have a problem with these things if this is what the family works out together, but it means so much more when it is parent and child creating the relationship for themselves rather than following a prescription.

I find, however, that the Lacanian process allows for that bond to occur as well, but is less directed and allows for more spontaneity and agency for the child. With children and our patients, we do not want to be the primary attachment figure. For some patients, I find I am that figure because the child does not have other attachment figures and is on family number ten. At some point, a lot of the work is about handing that over to the person who will be this child's family. This becomes about allowing space for the child to hand the primary attachment role over to someone else. I try to allow a space for a parent to be curious about their child. The parent is hopefully someone who is capable of that curiosity. Some parents may need a lengthy analysis to get there, but there are many people who are already there and are extraordinarily creative in coming up with ways to speak with their child. The parent may think of ways to connect with their child that I would never have thought and is far less formulaic.

CV: What was your motivation to do this kind of work?

KH: I enjoy working with young kids. I have a specialized thing insofar as working with children in foster care. I don't know at what moment I picked it, but I really like it. There is so much to think about. There is also something about the long-term nature of the work and all that can happen that I enjoy seeing. People will say about my work, "oh, how sad." My patients have been through horrible things, including trafficking and torture. People sometimes hear that and write off the child. What I enjoy being able to say is that no matter the history, I do not know what this child is going to do. I don't know what kind of life this child is going to make for themselves. To me, no matter how bad the history was, it does not necessarily determine anything about the child's future.

CV: Numerous times, someone or other has asked me what I do for a living. If I reply that I am a psychoanalyst, the person very often says some variation of the statement, "you must hear a lot of stories." I have heard this many times. I always wonder what the person is thinking in the moment when they say that. What does this person think I'm listening to? When someone says, "oh, how sad," to you, it is as if the statement actually says more about the person's fantasy of what is assumed to be the past of the child. When people say things like this about our work, it appears to be some fetishization of a dark history.

KH: It is the fetishization of trauma. I think that is something that Lacanian work does and should offer, that is, the lack of a fetishization of trauma, which means that a child has permission to be something other than their history. The door is always open for the child to pick things up in the direction that they choose. Sometimes I see foster and adoptive parents who tend to fetishize trauma. They want their child to be traumatized. It can be difficult. This is another way of talking about the symptom. The child comes in with symptoms of trauma because of what they went through and then at a certain point the child has to decide, "do I keep these symptoms for my adopted parents who want these?" or "do I let go of that and choose something else for myself?" It starts off as a series of events, but then it becomes something that someone else is very invested in.

I support this idea of trauma-informed schools. I talk to schools about being trauma-informed, which means to think about why a kid might be doing the stuff that they do. At the same time, I find that there becomes a troubling narrative around a kid who is traumatized as in that is who they are, and that is who they will be. There is not enough of a narrative about the potential to recover from trauma.

CV: Perhaps to transform it?

KH: Yes, or transcend it.

Note

1 This conversation took place on 8 April 2020.

Works Cited

Lacan, Jacques. "Les complexes familiaux dans la formation de l'individu: Essai d'analyse d'une function en psychologie." *Autre écrits*. Paris: aux Éditions du Seuil, 2001.23–84.

Lacan, Jacques. "Note sur l'enfant." *Autre écrits*. Paris: aux Éditions du Seuil, 2001.373–374.

Hennessy, Kristen. "From Edible to Oedipal: The Case of Jay." *Lacanian Psychoanalytic Technique Today*. Spec. issue of *Psychoanalytische Perspectieven*. 37.3 (2019): 829–837.

Hennessy, Kristen. "The Symptom and the System: Notes on the Foster Child." *Lacanian Psychoanalysis with Babies, Children, and Adolescents: Further Notes on the Child*. Ed. Carol Owens and Stephanie Farrelly Quinn. New York: Routledge, 2017.155–168.

Chapter 8

The Controlled Act of Psychotherapy in Ontario

A Lacanian Impasse

Sheila L. Cavanagh

> *From an analytic point of view, the only thing one can be guilty of is having given ground relative to one's desire.*
>
> (Lacan, *The Ethics of Psychoanalysis*, 319)

The 2007 Controlled Act of Psychotherapy is designed to regulate psychotherapy in Ontario. In 2017, the province proclaimed the act but granted a two-year transition period. Up until December 31, 2019, therapists could perform the Controlled Act of Psychotherapy so long as they did not call themselves psychotherapists while doing it. On January 1, 2020, the Act came into full force. Not only is the title controlled, but the psychotherapeutic act is now subject to legislative control. At the stroke of midnight, psychotherapy became a punishable act if not done in the right way, by the right person, with the right title, the right certification, the right authorization, the right restrictions governing treatment, and so on. All clinicians wishing to use the title "psychotherapist" or to commit the Controlled Act of Psychotherapy in the Canadian province must be registered by one of six regulatory Colleges of Ontario, qualifying for registration or a student in training.

What the province calls the controlled act of psychoanalysis surpasses governmental regulation in other jurisdictions (effectively making psychotherapy a criminal act) and is, as I will argue, at odds with what Jacques Lacan calls the psychoanalytic act. As he notes in his teachings, the psychoanalytic act is incongruous with the law and not amenable to control. As Lacan explains in his most important seminars related to the psychoanalytic act, *The Ethics of Psychoanalysis 1959–1960* (Book VII) and *The Psychoanalytic Act 1967–1968* (Book XV), the psychoanalytic act is transformative and particular to the subject. It cannot be prescribed or foreseen in advance. It concerns the desire and unconscious of the subject (as client). As such, the psychoanalytic act of concern to Lacanian psychoanalysis is incommensurate with a prescribed and mandated treatment protocol. It cannot be reconciled with regulatory compliance (the law), functionality (in the service

DOI: 10.4324/9781003212072-9

of capitalism, for example), positivity (happiness), or normalization. The psychoanalytic act cannot be controlled and is, in fact, a relinquishing of the significatory controls of the Other (as law or external agent).[1]

This is not a minor quibble. Nor is it superfluous when it comes to the question of psychoanalytic praxis. In fact, psychotherapeutic control is, for Lacan, precisely that which must be analyzed from the perspective of the analyst and abandoned. He tells those listening to his lecture of May 11, 1960: "At every moment we need to know what our effective relationship is to the desire to do good, to the desire to cure" (218), so as not to be led astray. Lacan is not making an argument against ethics but is, rather, skeptical about the way good intentions compromise psychoanalytic work with patients. Clinicians who follow Lacan must ask what kind of good the provincial legislation formalizes and if this good is in the best interests of clients (as desiring subjects). Lacan maintains that in order to do psychoanalysis, it may be necessary to refuse a "certain ideal of the good" that "erects a strong wall across the path of our desire. It is, in fact, at every moment and always, the first barrier that we have to deal with" (230). This chapter is guided by the Lacanian imperative to question the legal good for the greater psychoanalytic good of concern to ethical practice. Although Lacan theorizes many goods, utilitarian goods as distinct from the function of the beautiful (in the case of Antigone), the good that is promised to us without limit in what Lacan calls "the American way" (219), etc., I will, in this chapter, focus on the good concerning subjective desire. For Lacan, desire is the "metonymy of the discourse of demand" (*Seminar VII*, 293) that must be kept in motion. Desire takes the shape of a gap internal to the subject. It "insists on something else . . . beyond whatever it is able to formulate" (*Seminar VII*, 294) as demand.

In what follows, I discuss the Controlled Act of Psychotherapy in relation to Lacanian psychoanalytic ethics as related to accidents (and to what Louis Matheou (2018) calls *act*cidents), the linguistic operation (as distinct from a medical intervention), fantasy, the semblance, the Thing (*Das Ding*), acting out (in the repetition), and a passage to the act (the end goal and aim of psychoanalysis).

The CRPO and the Controlled Act of Psychotherapy

The Psychotherapy Act and the Regulated Health Professions Act (RHPA) authorizes the College of Registered Psychotherapists of Ontario (CRPO)[2] to regulate psychotherapy.[3] The CRPO has the legislative authority to define what counts as psychotherapy (under the auspices of the controlled act), to regulate the practice and all titles affiliated with psychotherapy. Schedule R, section 11 of *The Psychotherapy Act* gives the College council permission to "make regulations prescribing therapies involving the practice of psychotherapy, governing the use of prescribed therapies and prohibiting the use of therapies other than the prescribed therapies in the course of the practice of psychotherapy".[4] The CRPO council has the authority to investigate and discipline practitioners who may be operating unlawfully under the title "psychotherapist," to mandate professional training consistent with best practices as they define them, to impose fines for violations of College rules, to regulate training, licensing, etc., in the name of the "public good."

The Controlled Act of Psychotherapy should give all clinicians, Lacanian and otherwise, cause for concern from a legal and ethical standpoint. I will begin with the law. From a legal perspective, the Psychotherapy Act is anomalous and posits a false correspondence between a medical and psychotherapeutic intervention. The act is anomalous, in part, because no other province or territory in Canada has (at the time of writing) comparable legislation.[5] Nor is there a comparable international example whereby psychotherapy is criminalized in addition to being regulated. There is a critical difference between "regulations" and "controlled acts" under the RHPA. Regulation is done through licensing and accreditation processes established by governing bodies in order to protect the public. There are legitimate arguments to be made for the regulation of psychotherapy, but controlling psychotherapy is another matter entirely. It is one thing to revoke one's license to practice, to refuse membership to a regulatory College, to hold providers to account for malpractice, to investigate complaints relating to sexual boundary violations, etc. But it is another thing to control the act of psychotherapy, thereby making it a criminal offense. It should be noted that the Health Professions Regulatory Advisory Council (HPRAC) recommended regulation of psychotherapy to the Minister, but not control. In 2006, the Council submitted their extensive report, entitled *Regulation of Health Professionals in Ontario: New Directions* to the Minister. Following a year of expansive consultation with almost 2000 "health professionals, associations, regulatory colleges and hundreds of individuals" (1), the HPRAC advised George Smitherman, Minister of Health and Long-Term Care, not to control the act of psychotherapy:

> The disadvantage is that it would require a precise definition of the act of psychotherapy comparable to the wording of the 13 existing controlled acts under the statute. This is not viable, because psychotherapy is a process and cannot be characterized as a single act.
>
> (217)

Against HPRAC advice, the Minister made psychotherapy a controlled act. The College of Physicians and Surgeons of Ontario (CPSO) seems to be in agreement with the HPRAC's initial recommendation. They issued a statement to the government whereby they explain that the risk of harm to clients referred to in the act is "technically inaccurate" and does not "align with the medical model" whereby acts are controlled.[6] HPRAC also wrote (in a later document) that CPSO pulled out of a working group convened by the CRPO to review issues associated with the legislation. The document, entitled "Understanding When Psychotherapy is a Controlled Act" (June 2016), also referred to as the "Clarification Document" (to the MOHLTC), was endorsed by all regulatory Colleges in Ontario except CPSO.

Like CPSO, the Ontario Public Service Employees Union (OPSEU) explains that "the medical model does not easily translate to community-based services." By making psychotherapy a controlled act, the province is comparing a therapeutic conversation to an objective medical intervention. Controlled acts in Ontario have, until recently, included medical procedures like surgeries and other physical interventions. Medical acts are controlled to protect the public from gross negligence and malpractice leading to physical injury. There are 14 controlled acts in Ontario. They include: communications relating to diagnosis; medical procedures such as setting (casting) a bone fracture; moving spinal joints; the administration of controlled substances; inserting instruments, hands, or fingers in bodily cavities; ordering or applying energy; prescribing, dispensing, or selling drugs; the prescription of hearing aids; fitting or dispensing dental appliances and devices; managing the delivery of a baby; allergy testing; and now (wait for it) *psychotherapy*.

As the iconic song by Joe Raposo and Jon Stone (made famous on the 1970s children's television show *Sesame Street*) goes, "One of These Things Is Not Like the Others." At risk of stating the obvious, it is psychotherapy. I do not wish to undermine the seriousness of the psychotherapeutic enterprise or to cast dispersion on policy advisors, legislators, and members of the CRPO who may believe they are doing a public service. Nor do I suggest that people cannot be hurt by psychotherapy. But it does not follow that psychotherapy is synonymous with a medical intervention. Nor should it be a criminal offense. Controlling medical acts mitigates against mistakes made by unlicensed providers: accidents that can cause irreversible physical harm, even death. Although accidents happen in the clinic of psychotherapy, these accidents are of a different order relating to what is often called the therapeutic alliance. This does not make them less serious, but it does make them more complicated. For one, the harm engendered in the clinic of psychotherapy is not always or, perhaps, exclusively detrimental to the client. Of course, a sexual boundary violation is harmful and not analytically productive, but mistakes made by client and psychotherapist alike are of a different magnitude and significance. In fact, harm may be an unavoidable part of the cure. Sometimes psychotherapeutic work deepens when a clinical mistake is made and acknowledged and becomes a point of dialogue. It is important to distinguish between an abuse of professional power and the mistakes, let us call them accidents, that clinical work may depend upon. In *Seminar XVIII*, Lacan contends that the passage to the act is an accident. It is not an intention and cannot be controlled. It may only be understood in the Afterward (*après-coup*). One way to illustrate the difference between harm caused by malpractice and an associated abuse of professional power, and harm, including clinical mistakes, that are part of the human experience and, by extension, all relationships, including psychotherapeutic relationships (as defined by the CRPO), is to consider the difference between accidents and *act*cidents (Matheou 2018).

Psychotherapeutic *Act*cidents and Accidents

Louis Matheou (2018) offers a discussion of the actcident in Lacanian psychoanalytic ethics. Accidents are to be distinguished from the *act*cidents of concern to not only victims of medical malpractice suits but also clients subject to, for instance, professional boundary violations in the psychotherapy clinic. *Act*cidents are, unlike accidents, intentional. *Act*cidents occur when elements of subjectivity, including speech, are foreclosed. The provincial legislation governing psychotherapy is actcidental because it outlaws a form of speech central to Lacanian psychoanalytic practice. *Act*cidents occur when speech is delimited by external agents. The signifiers of relevance to the psychotherapist and client alike are overdetermined by legal agents, rendered mum, or, in Lacanian terms, foreclosed when subjects relating to desire, as opposed to diagnosis, are rendered irrelevant or at odds with best practice.

When, for instance, the spontaneous speech of the analysand is subject to the delineation and inscription of a presenting problem (diagnosis), incorporated into an agreed upon case-formulation in the first session (or two) (template-based session notes), treated through CRPO protocols, diagnosed and evaluated in terms of impairment (functionality), seriousness (by whose estimate we are not sure), etc., the client-analysand cannot say anything new, anything of relevance to the particularity of their experience. Nothing that has not already been subject to regulatory control can be thought or said, let alone done in the name of psychotherapy. This is not a minor problem from a psychoanalytic perspective. As Lacan says, it concerns the linguistic operation of concern to the analytic cure. The ethic of psychoanalysis is about the desire of the subject and the difficult task of enabling the subject to speak. But this is not any kind of speech. Lacan is concerned with a particular way of speaking relevant to the question of desire. In Lacan's very first seminar, "Freud's Papers on Technique: 1953–1954," he says that "an act is speech" (246). This is not to say that speech *is* an act but, rather, that the psychoanalytic act takes the form of speech. It is a subjective declaration of sorts. The speech is unique and particular to the analytic subject.

The *Controlled Act of Psychotherapy* does not enable analytic speech. In fact, it precludes it. Everything that can be said and heard is assimilated into an assessment tool and reduced to an indicator of an already imagined diagnosis or impairment. Nothing can be heard in the controlled clinic that is not an indicator of a mental health diagnosis, impairment, or dysfunction. Desire is irrelevant. The signifier cannot act when everything has been overwritten by treatment protocols regulated by the CRPO. As Lacan explains, "a signifying organization dominates the psychic apparatus as it is revealed to us in the examination of a patient" (*Seminar VII*, 118). It is there, in the signifying system, that the linguistic operation of concern to Lacanian psychoanalysis must occur. But the diagnostic and measurement tools provided by the HPRAC (2017, 15) petrify speech. The signifier of concern to the psychotherapeutic dyad is mummified. This not only thwarts the analytic endeavor but, from a Lacanian view, also harms the client.

Unlike an accident, which can be analytically productive in the form of Freudian slips, parapraxes, and so forth, the actcident misfires in psychoanalytically unhelpful ways. When Freud talks about parapraxes, he is not talking about incompetence or negligence on the part of clinicians, but rather about how we may learn something about the unconscious by attending to the analysand's accidents (at the level of speech). *Act*cidents, for Matheou (2018), preclude subjective responsibility. When clinical acts are *act*cidental the subject is left unchanged, unable to assume a subjective presence in the face of the Other (of the Symbolic), unable to act psychoanalytically. Nothing can happen to the *act*cidental subject. The subject is not only defended but also over-determined by the Other's desire in me. This is an *act*cident subject to repetition. The subject-analysand cannot assume responsibility for a cure, with and alongside an analyst, when the Other (as law) overshadows the work. The subject needs to work through the way they are "immersed in the pre-given" (Matheou 2018): in what Lacan calls the law and desire of the Other.

The psychoanalytic act is precisely what would enable the subject to liberate themselves from the law, desire, and demand of the Other and to assume responsibility. If the Controlled Act of Psychotherapy is, in fact, an actcident, psychoanalysis, let alone psychotherapy, will be compromised. But this is not all. Lacanian practice attends not only to desire, to the speaking subject, but also to *jouissance*. *Jouissance* is a French term Lacan uses to interpret something beyond what Freud calls the pleasure principle: something that is not only exciting and painful, but too much. Addictions, for instance, can be *jouissant*. *Jouissance* bothers and excites the subject. We might say that jouissance causes harm. But it is a harm (akin to what Lacan calls a "little death" in orgasm) that we cannot, as subjects of language, forgo. We are all beings toward death in Freudian and Lacanian terms. This is a difficult psychoanalytic truth.

For Matheou, the "*act*cident is an act in which the death drive meets with a traumatic incidence that results both in the death and continued survival of the subject" (2018, 341). Matheou is talking about a life devoid of desire and the capacity to act. Just like Antigone (in the Sophocles play by the same name), who does not relent upon her desire to bury her brother in Theban soil (despite the threat of death issued by the King), the client whose desire cannot be heard in the actcidental clinic must endure a little death. In other words, something of significance relating to their experience will be eclipsed. In non-Lacanian terms, we might say that the client will be unheard and hurt again by a Registered Psychotherapist (RP) who adheres to the letter of the law, as opposed to the words of concern to the client's experience. Much like the Controlled Act of Psychotherapy envisions a client-subject who can be cured (or at least relieved) of psychiatric distress, impairments, dysfunctions, and so forth, the actcidental subject of concern to Matheou (2018) is without lack (and thus desire). In other words, both subjects are erroneously imagined, or imposed upon, to be symptom-free. From a Lacanian standpoint, this is fraudulent. No one can be post-traumatic, that is, without a symptom. Like a signature, a symptom authenticates our being in the place of an impasse.

But it is tempting to regard one's clients as symptom-free or to treat them as if they will one day be symptom-free (that is, post-traumatic) when the weight of the law is hanging overhead. The bonds of the law are not easily broken. It is not for nothing that Lacan uses the writings of the Marquis de Sade to illustrate the way we are tethered to the law and suffer accordingly. Clients do, say, feel, and conceal things we do not want to hear. If the psychotherapy clinic cannot be a place to hear difficult things about the human experience, things that are, have been, and will continue to be hurtful, negative and at odds with the discourse of mental hygiene, there will be no psychoanalysis as Lacan understood it. If clinical notes are to be subject to sporadic reviews by the CRPO, ready for subpoena by the courts, suitable for review by insurance companies, etc., they will not be composed of analytic material relating to desire and *jouissance*, to the imperceptible "Thing" haunting the client. Clinician notes will be sanitized of all relevant psychoanalytic material. If a client persists in expressing symptoms that appear to be disordered, indicative of impairments, dysfunctionality, and so on, they will be dropped (or referred elsewhere) by RPs. Unregulated providers will also be less likely to take these clients on because they are now liable to be accusations of unlawfully committing the controlled Act if they work with clients who may be classified as "disordered" or "impaired."[7]

The College and provincial legislation authorizing it may, in the spirit of the public good, do no harm, but they will also do no, or very little, good for those most in need of psychotherapeutic support. While Lacan insists that the analysand is the only one who acts (in psychoanalytic terms), the legislation places responsibility for the act on the provider (analyst). Many therapists in Ontario are, consequently, afraid of the legislation and wondering, with good reason, if they may be liable to a fine up to $25,000 for a first offence, and up to $50,000 for a second offence. According to Schedule R of the Act, such fines may also be coupled with imprisonment for up to a year. Unregulated therapists are now likely to refuse work with at-risk clients, including those with a psychiatric diagnosis, because they are now vulnerable to criminal charges. Volunteers are also less likely to work as counsellors for Ontario's frontline mental health support services for fear of breaking a law that is based on imprecise terms of reference.[8]

The Linguistic Operation and the Medical Scalpel

In Lacanian psychoanalysis, the linguistic operation that occurs in analysis is not equivalent to the work undertaken by a surgeon who uses, among other things, a medical scalpel. This may seem obvious, but the provincial legislation equates the two. The Controlled Act of Psychotherapy is predicated upon the assumption that what happens in analysis is comparable to what happens in a medical environment. The controlled act is, in other words, analogous to medical procedures, including but not limited to surgeries. The psychoanalytic act operates at the level of discourse for Lacan. Although the psychoanalyst targets the signifier of concern to the analysand, their intervention is guided by the client. A critical difference can be seen in the way a medical doctor determines the nature and course of a physical intervention, whereas an analyst cannot know, let alone determine in advance, what type of scansion will take route in the unconscious. A medical procedure is more likely to be unidirectional and led, if not wholly determined, by a medical professional.

Unlike a Lacanian analyst who engages the subject of language, the medical doctor engages the subject of physiology. While there is a relationship, albeit a complicated one, between the signifying body and the corporeal body in Lacanian psychoanalysis, they should not be conflated in one fell legislative swoop. There are differences between the way the signifier acts on the body in psychotherapy and the way a medical scalpel cuts into anaesthetized bodies. The subjective and objective operate on different levels, although they intersect each of the three Lacanian psychic registers (the Symbolic, the Imaginary, and the Real). A signifier acts on each register in Lacanian terms, but not like an epidermic needle. Lacanian psychoanalysts may puncture a patient's discourse and, in so doing, inject a question, isolate, or accentuate a signifier to alter the subject's relation to the Other. But this is altogether different from a medical injection or drawing blood with a lancet device.

Moreover, physicians do not routinely establish relationships with their clients, at least not therapeutic relationships, unless, of course, they are monitoring medications or combining psychiatric work with psychotherapy in their practice. But even then, the relationships are usually structured by the physician and not led by the client. Certainly, there are medical doctors in the province who are also psychoanalysts and psychotherapists, but my point is that medical procedures subject to legal control are not equivalent to psychotherapy. This is not to say that a medical intervention cannot have an impact upon how a patient feels about themselves, upon their subjective experience as such. A patient may feel differently after a spinal joint is adjusted or a hearing aid inserted into the ear cavity. It is not uncommon for patients to attribute meaning to medical procedures in the afterward. A medical act can have what Lacan calls a signifying effect, but this effect is secondary and not intentional. The intention of a medically controlled act is not to engage unconscious processes. Although doctors, like all medical professionals, talk to their patients (and bedside manner is important), the intervention itself does not usually require talk, let alone a psychotherapeutic relationship as defined by the CRPO.[9]

As most psychoanalysts will agree, the analytic relationship is unlike any other relationship, including those between a medical doctor and a patient. In Lacanian terms, there is always a third (an Other) in any given psychoanalytic dyad: the analyst, the analysand, and the Other of the unconscious (which includes the law, language, and the Symbolic). A medical procedure may involve actual others like, for instance, nurses and occupational therapists, but the Other of the unconscious is not needed to initiate the procedure. A root canal cannot be compared to the scansion of a signifier at the level of speech. Certainly, the client's unconscious is not on a dental hygienist's mind when cleaning a patient's teeth. Although Freud wrote much about the oral stage, oral eroticism, and oral fixations in those weaned from the mother's breast too early, this phase of psychosexual development is not relevant to dentistry as a profession.

Regardless of our view on the psychotherapeutic relationship, its composition and relation to the unconscious, the research is clear. The only reliable indicator of a successful psychotherapeutic treatment is in the strength of the therapeutic alliance. The therapeutic alliance, like any relationship (regardless of its status as a legal entity), is not something that flourishes in controlled environments. As any feminist psychotherapist will tell you, a relationship ceases to be a relationship when it is subject to control, let alone regulation and governance. But more than this, a relationship, in Lacanian terms, involves fantasy (among other things). A relationship works when it is animated by something operating at the level of fantasy (which Lacan likens to *object a*). For Lacan, a non-object causes desire and enables something akin to a relationship to occur. We do not know and relate to others in the ways we think we do. We relate to the object cause of our own desire (appearing in the orbit of the Other), to something fantastical beyond signification, and not to others in particular. The impasse between speaking subjects thus informs the clinical relationship. If a relationship is to work (which is different from positing its existence as such), it will, as Lacan explains in his seminar on the *sinthome* (an old term for symptom), do so in the place of an impasse. That is to say, the psychoanalytic relationship (if we can agree to call it that) occurs in the place of a gap or impasse between speaking subjects. There is no understanding the other in Lacanian psychoanalysis. Rather, there is a focus upon what cannot be understood at the level of fantasy (the Real). The analytic relationship works when there is an intervention at the level of fantasy, not at the level of the intersubjective relationship (contra relational psychoanalysis).

Despite the impact of the psychotherapeutic alliance (however we might understand it psychoanalytically), it does not carry physical risks akin to medical procedures. Unlike psychotherapists, surgeons operate on the body without attention to the signifier, the discourse of the patient. A surgeon, like an anesthesiologist or a dentist, intervenes at the level of the actual physical body almost exclusively. If they cut an artery by mistake, a patient may die. The medical professional acts to save lives, to cast a bone fracture, to apply a dental prosthetic, to palliate physical (as opposed to psychosomatic) suffering by medication, etc. There are risks associated with these procedures that are different and more serious than those likely to occur in the clinic of psychotherapy. At risk of stating the obvious, psychotherapy is unlikely to kill a patient in the way a cut artery, an overdose, a drug prescription, or injection can. It makes sense that these medical acts are subject to legislative control. No one (to my knowledge) has overdosed, bled to death, or had an allergic reaction to a conversation with a psychotherapist. This is not to say that a psychotherapist cannot cause harm to a client or that boundary violations do not occur, including, but not limited to, sexual boundary violations, breaches of confidentiality, and so forth. It is, however, to suggest that these risks are more likely to be mitigated by regulation than control.

Does the Controlled Act of Psychotherapy Exist?

The Controlled Act of Psychotherapy is, unlike other controlled acts in the province regulated by the RHPA, causing confusion and fear. It causes fear in counsellors and unregulated providers who do not want to be accused of committing the controlled act (beyond their legal scope of practice), but no one seems to know what exactly it is in clinical practice. Yet, unregulated providers are responsible for assessing whether or not they are, or could be, committing a Controlled Act of Psychotherapy. Nobody really knows what the act is in practice, if they can do it, if they are doing it without authorization, if it can be restricted, and what the legal consequences will be should they become a test-case.[10] The legislation lacks precision, and unregulated providers are put into legally precarious positions. Unregistered providers – those who are counsellors and, by the CRPO's own admission, provide valuable and important services to clients – are at legal risk. Unregistered therapists, counsellors, and other mental health service providers cannot differentiate what they do from what they must not do because the difference between psychotherapy in general and the Controlled Act of Psychotherapy cannot be substantiated in clinical practice. Even the province seems to know that the legislation is ill-defined, and the CRPO is attempting to delineate the act more clearly.[11] But this delineation will always be precarious in practice because the subjective elements of psychotherapies are Real (beyond signification) and cannot be legally circumscribed or defined to anyone's satisfaction. Let us consider the function of the act and the legal definition to illustrate my point.

The Controlled Act of Psychotherapy in Ontario is defined in the *Regulated Health Professions Act* as "treating, by means of psychotherapy technique, delivered through a therapeutic relationship, an individual's serious disorder of thought, cognition, mood, emotional regulation, perception or memory that may seriously impair the individual's judgement, insight, behavior, communication or social functioning." The Act includes a focus on diagnosis, impairment, outcomes, predetermined goals, and plans, along with clear distinctions between beginnings and endings. If an unregistered clinician discovers that they are committing the act of psychotherapy, they are legally required to restrict their practice or to join one of the five Colleges recognized by the *Regulated Health Professions Act*.[12]

In essence, the legislation makes a particular scope of practice internal to psychotherapy a controlled act. But the key words in the act are, like all signifiers, slippery. The five components of the Act relating to the psychotherapeutic treatment, technique, relationship, and seriousness of the relevant disorder and impairment treated are all imprecise and ill-defined. I am not the only one to notice this.[13] No one knows for certain what counts as a "disorder," as an "impairment," as "serious," as a "psychotherapy technique," as a "therapeutic relationship," etc., in clinical terms. Moreover, the general (unregulated) components of psychotherapy are not discernable from the scope of practice subject to legislative control. Even those clinicians accepting of the psychiatric language of disorders and diagnosis incorporated into the act will have questions. Are there unserious disorders and impairments? Must a client be assessed by a psychiatrist to be designated disordered (and impaired), or can they be disordered (and impaired) in the absence of a psychiatric diagnosis? What if a provider does their due diligence by completing an intake assessment and the client does not disclose a history of depression, for instance? Let us presume that the provider and client agree that the presenting problem is ambivalence, chronic indecision (not depression), and then each party discovers retroactively that what they thought was ambivalence is, from a psychiatric perspective, depression? Does it matter that the client does not think they are depressed? Would the provider be guilty of treating depression, a serious disorder, all along in such a case? What if the client has a psychiatric diagnosis but disidentifies with the diagnosis, preferring instead to view their symptom-set as neurodiverse and unproblematic? Let us presume that an unregistered clinician agrees to work with such a client, restricts their practice (as advised by the College), does not hold themselves out as a RP, and acts to the best of their ability in accordance with the law – would they be at risk of contravening the Act?

Even the CRPO cannot answer these questions. But this does not stop the proliferation of materials designed to further regulate and control psychotherapy by making the act visible. According to the province, the controlled scope of practice, relevant to the Psychotherapy Act (2007), involves five subsidiary components that are to be made visible and thus identifiable. For example, in a clarification document issued by the HPRA, it says that the "key elements of this [psychotherapy] relationship are [to be] observable by both the provider and the client" (2017, 6). This is a strange injunction. Unlike a flayed corpse made visible to a surgical team during an operation, a psychotherapist cannot make a client's psychology visible. Nor can a relationship be observable. We can make inferences about the therapeutic alliance, but these inferences are interpretations and thus subjective, not objective. Subjective phenomenon, unlike the physical environment, cannot be subject to empirical validation by sight. I dare say we have all had the experience of thinking a relationship, therapeutic or otherwise, was going well, that progress was being made (whatever that might mean), only to discover retroactively that the other person had a completely different understanding of what was occurring in the imagined relationship. Other worldly galaxies, including the rights of Saturn, can be made visible through a telescope. But even planetary scientists will concede that there is a difference between what is seen and the actual planetary phenomenon subject to observation.

I cannot help but wonder if the Controlled Act of Psychotherapy is requiring providers to participate in a collective delusion whereby they must claim to see things, to make elements of their practice empirical or visible, that are not ocular. But even if a provider imagines they know what the controlled act is in clinical practice and that they can make it visible to clients (as they are told they must by the CRPO), they will have to negotiate an impasse between what the law says they are, or must be, doing and what their clients think they are, or should be, doing. Consider a client who comes to psychotherapy for a better understanding of why they are unhappy at work, why they seek out lovers who hurt them, what, if anything, they can do about the deleterious effects of anti-black racism, the way intergenerational traumas dating back to the Canadian residential school system affect their native identity, the existential uncertainties of life in what environmentalists call the Anthropocene, etc., and the psychotherapist who is trained to focus on the assessment of disorders, impairments, and dysfunctions in those schools, institutes, and universities accredited by the CRPO as separate from politics.[14] The psychotherapist registered with the CRPO has a difficult ethical choice to make. Do they tell the client that psychotherapy is not about the philosophies of life (as understood by Socrates or Indigenous healers, for instance), Eros (involving, among other things, the question of desire), the impact of white settler colonialism on the suffering of Indigenous peoples, the depressing effects of the neo-liberal capitalist workplace, the reality of global climate warming, etc., but rather about the way they, as client, are disordered, impaired, and dysfunctional? In other words, does the RP posit a false separation between the individual-subject (as client) and society (the Other of language, law, culture and so forth)? In so doing, would the RP not be inadvertently blaming the client for their inability to accommodate to the institutions of late, modern, industrial, capitalist, western settler colonialism? A psychotherapist does not have to be Lacanian (or overtly political) to recognize that the disorders and impairments said to be serious in the act do not occur in a vacuum. The correlation between trauma and psychiatric disorders, impairments, addictions, and so forth are significant and should not be sidelined. I imagine the regulators would counter that there is, in fact, a wide range of therapeutic space of practice to maneuver outside the inner circle of the controlled act, that they are only regulating a tiny scope within the larger domain of psychotherapy. This may be true in theory and on paper. But let us remember that a client does not check their diagnosis at the clinical door. Even if a client comes to see a counsellor for career or educational advice, feelings of anxiety and depression (often said, or later found, to be serious) will often emerge. I cannot imagine anyone, regardless of their psychological resiliency, being entirely without anxiety and depression. We should pause to ask when and how therapy became the domain of psychiatry (and pharmacology), as opposed to philosophy, sociology, and even religion. Fortunately, the act exempts Indigenous healers in the province, but there are multiple other spiritual practices dating back to antiquity that may provide important therapeutic counters to what Bulgarian psychoanalyst Julia Kristeva calls the new maladies of the soul in her book by the same name (1995).

There are, by the HPRACC's own count, over 200 forms of psychotherapy (2017, 41). These therapeutic approaches, despite their effectiveness, will, over time, disappear or become rare in the controlled environment. The CRPO now accredits psychotherapy training programs in the province. The curriculum, clinical practice, and supervision are all subject to the approval of the College. Only those psychotherapy training programs that adopt textbooks and approaches to psychotherapy predicated upon psychology (usually cognitive behavioral therapy (CBT) or Dialectical Behavior Therapy (DBT)), as opposed to, for example, holistic healing, art therapy, Jungian psychology, psychoanalysis, etc., are approved by the CRPO (unless, of course, they make these "alternative" approaches secondary to the reigning methods of psychology). Even the psychoanalytic institutes in Toronto that have long traditions of respecting unconscious processes in their teachings, supervision, and clinical work are shifting their programs to more psychiatric and ego-psychology models.

The reduction of therapy to individual psychology is a distinctly modern phenomenon that Lacan, in his critique of American ego-psychology, railed against in his teachings. In Lacanian psychoanalysis and, also, in

trauma-informed approaches to psychotherapy, the individual is not imagined to be separable from the Other (of society). Individual psychologies do not take shape independent of the external environment. One's experience of the Other (and otherness) is intimately linked to the very symptoms subject to assessment. When psychotherapists are imposed upon to focus on the individual and not the Other (inclusive of the law, language, and the Symbolic), analytic work is thwarted. The Lacanian registers call upon us to imagine a continuum between the subject (as client) and the Other. From a Lacanian perspective, psychotherapeutic practice (in general) and the Controlled Act of Psychotherapy (the inner circle) are homeomorphic.

That is to say that they are continuous functions and, in essence, the same. If there is a difference between what is inside the enclosure (the Controlled Act of Psychotherapy) and outside the enclosure (psychotherapy in general), it is unstable and intermeshed. Perhaps a better way to illustrate the non-differential relation between psychotherapy in general and the controlled act in particular is to say that they are isomorphic (inverse mappings of identical structures). Lacan used knot-theory and complex geometry to demonstrate the human psyche for a reason. Psychotherapy, like the human psyche, is not two-dimensional. Human subjectivity is multidimensional and better represented as a Möbius strip (where what is inside meets the outside, and what is outside meets the inside). The difference between the inner circle (subject to legislative control) and the outer circle (open to unregulated providers) is not only illusory but also legally and clinically untenable.

The Thing (*Das Ding*)

Most people will agree that there is something about the human experience that assessment tools focused upon diagnosis, impairments, etc., miss. Lacan calls this thing *das Ding*, a German word he adopts to refer to the unconscious "Thing" lacking symbolization. *Das Ding* (or the Thing) in the Lacanian lexicon refers to something that occurs in the register of the Real (the psychic register beyond signification). It is also used by Lacan in his later work to refer to the object of desire (*object a*), a primordial Other or lost-object that cannot be had or found. Although the Thing of concern to Lacan does not appear as such, it causes desire. It is, to use a contemporary colloquialism, *not a thing*: it is the Thing.

In *Seminar VII*, where Lacan devotes a year to the ethics of psychoanalysis, he focuses on the gap between the subject and the mysterious Thing (which he later equates with "a" from 1963 onwards). The Thing (which Lacan also calls *das Ding*) is "attached to whatever is open, lacking, or gaping at the center of our desire" (*Seminar VII*, 84). It is distinct from the object. The Thing is, for Lacan, "what in the real suffers from the signifier" (*Seminar VII*, 125). It is thus a catalyst for desire. As such, it must not be filled. We may try to find the Thing, in Freudian terms, but it is "to be found at the most as something missed. One doesn't find it, but only its pleasurable associations" (*Seminar VII*, 52).

We might imagine the gap of concern to Lacan to resonate with a feeling of internal emptiness. For others, the gap may be intercepted as something that we miss or cannot attain, again (like a repetition). Lacks and gaps in the client's discourse relating to what cannot be said concerning, for instance, a traumatic event, must be analyzed at the level of the signifier if the client is going to alter their relation to the traumatic event. Lacan contends that anxiety emerges when the gap or lack in being foundational to the subject is threatened. But no matter how we understand the lack in being or the Thing that causes desire, there is, for Lacan, a gap that must be maintained.

My concern is that the Act is foreclosing upon the space and possibility of the psychoanalytic act as understood by Lacan, predicated as it is upon a subjective (and interpersonal) gap. CRPO regulators do not want to know anything about the unconscious, let alone the gap of concern to Lacanian psychoanalysts. The appearance of something psychotherapeutic is what, ultimately, matters to the College. From a Lacanian perspective, we may understand the Controlled Act of Psychotherapy to be a semblant. A semblant (like a faulty sign) directs us away from a void. It acts to camouflage a lack in being. The Lacanian semblant, like the Act, is deceptive. The semblant plays with appearances. Much like the controlled act conceals an unbearable truth relating to the clinic of psychotherapy, the semblant is an illusion. In the context of legislative control, the semblant masks what cannot be objectively seen in the psychotherapeutic method itself. The Lacanian semblant is a substitute for a primary object. Likewise, the controlled act is a substitute for something more psychoanalytically significant, something irreducible to the discourse of the law adopted by regulators. Legislators and regulators do not like to acknowledge that there is something about the psychotherapeutic relationship that cannot be seen, let alone controlled. It is hard to accept that psychotherapy is not an objective science. Psychotherapy defies objective measure but when it works, the subjective effects are incalculable.

Psychotherapy cannot be controlled because we cannot say with any degree of certainty what happens between therapist and client, what transpires to enable or disable, a cure at the level of the transference. Perhaps we can agree on elements relating to the psychotherapeutic frame including, for instance, a 50-minute session, an agreed upon fee schedule, session dates and times, and so forth (despite Lacan's refusal to maintain a standard frame). But the frame is not the psychotherapeutic act. It is meant to enable it. Unlike the frame, the traumata revealed in the transference (what the client projects on to the psychoanalyst) cannot be observed, let alone controlled.

Despite this, regulators want evidence of effectivity and quality assurance. Equally, clients do not want to know that the outcomes of psychotherapy cannot be assured or that what bothers them may also cause them to desire and to be as subjects of language. When entering into a therapeutic relationship, clients want to know they are getting the real thing (not charlatans). Clinicians wanting to do right by their clients also seek quality assurance. No one wants to be a bad therapist, the therapist who does not do *it* or get *it*. In their early days of practice, it is not uncommon for therapists to seek reassurance from supervisors. The new clinician wants to know if they are doing *it* (that is, psychotherapy) right. Is something happening or not?

The demand for psychotherapeutic visibility, accountability, and efficacy is widespread. But this demand conceals a more fundamental truth relating to the unquantifiability of the therapeutic endeavor. Clinicians may, like agents of the law, take comfort in the illusion that something in the name of psychotherapy can be affirmed like an event. But the quality assurance is temporary at best. Like all defenses it comes up short. I wager a guess that all psychotherapists (registered or not) in Ontario wake up at night with a niggling suspicion that the Act is a red herring and, as such, a semblant, an appearance of something where there is, in fact, nothing.

Acting Out: Recognition, Demand, and Plagiarism in the Professional Transference

From a Lacanian standpoint, I wonder if the legislation is not a transferential act. In other words, I wonder if, in controlling the act of psychotherapy along with psychotherapists subject to it, the College and the legislators who authorize it are acting out. Acting out has a special meaning in Lacanian psychoanalysis. Acting out is, in Freudian and Lacanian terms, about being caught in the transference. It functions as an obstacle to the psychoanalytic act. The nature and type of enactment, repetitive as it is, helps us to understand what needs to be done, what resistances need to be overcome. One acts out what cannot be remembered. As such, the act replaces speech. While it may, in Freudian terms, be resistance, the acting out is, for Lacan, a message in disguise. In *Seminar V*, Lacan describes "acting out" as a message relating to a problem between desire and demand.

Acting out is a demand made to the Other for recognition. In the clinic, the analysand who acts out is operating in the transference. As such, they make a demand of the analyst as subject supposed to know. Acting out, in Lacanian terms, can also be read as a refusal of castration (which involves the way we are cut by language). We are trapped in a network of signifiers. In acting out, one refuses, or tries to refuse, alienation (castration) by the signifier. For Lacan, a signifier represents a subject for another signifier. As such, it will not stay put. The signifier does not have a definitive meaning but, nevertheless, constitutes the subject of the unconscious. Unlike a sign (which has a meaning for Lacan), a signifier does not produce a unifying meaning for the subject. While every subject has a master signifier, no signifier can ever, finally, represent the subject split (as we all are) by language. Acting out produces what Owen Hewitson calls, in his discussion of *Seminar III* on *LacanOnline*, a "hastily provided symbolization, like that found in what are known as the 'elementary phenomena' of psychosis" ("Acting Out").

While I will save the question of psychotic legislation for another day, the College does have an obsession with significatory titles: their use, restriction, and authorization. In keeping with the Controlled Act of Psychotherapy, the title "psychotherapist" is restricted. As per a 2009 amendment to the Psychotherapy Act, only members of the CRPO may use the title "RP" or a "variation or abbreviation or an equivalent in another language." Members cannot use a "name other than the member's name as entered in the register" or use a "term, title or designation indicating or implying a specialization in the profession" inappropriately. Psychotherapists must use the titles designated by the College while "acting in a professional capacity." Others are not legally entitled to "hold himself or herself out as a person who is qualified to practice in Ontario" (Psychotherapy Act, 2007, SO 2007, c 10, Sch R).

Protected titles relating to psychotherapy are not only creating a new professional identity politic enforced by the Colleges but are also indicative of a larger problem with what Sigmund Freud calls "the narcissism of minor differences" (*Civilization and Its Discontents* 69). The greatest identitarian battles are fought between people, groups, communities, nations, etc., who have the most in common. Counsellors and psychotherapists, RPs and unregulated psychotherapists have a lot in common. The legal politics governing professional titles are said to be about public protection, but I wonder if they are not more about controlling professional jurisdiction, establishing a monopoly, and managing liability. There is no evidence to suggest that the public is better served by registered than by unregistered clinicians. It can also not be said that RPs have more clinical experience than unregistered psychotherapists. It is, however, true that RPs are more likely to have training and clinical hours compliant with CRPO requirements. But compliance does not produce better psychotherapists. It produces psychotherapists with training, supervision, and clinical hours approved by the CRPO and thus in compliance with the psycho-medical model.

Compliance enables a clinician to use and access protected titles like, for instance, RP. If a client has a psychotherapist with an authorized title, they are "protected" from unregulated providers, counsellors, coaches, etc., posing as "real" psychotherapists. The public does not know that many of Ontario's unregulated providers have more and diversified clinical experience than the newly minted RPs in the province. Let us also be clear about the fact that most clients do not understand the difference between a Registered Psychotherapist (RP), a Qualifying Psychotherapist (QP), or an unregulated psychotherapist until they consult their insurance plan or submit a claim for reimbursement for therapy. Even when a client is aware of their provider's registration status and title, it does not alter or affect the course of therapy unless a lack of registration causes the client to question the legitimacy of the clinician. Lacan explains that the analyst must be the one supposed to know, not the one actually in the know. It is much better if the analyst does not know or keeps what they think they know out of the analytic equation in Lacan's view. This is not an argument against psychoanalytic interpretation, education, and supervised clinical practice but more a commentary on how it is better to be curious about a client than to presume to know anything, in particular, about a client. Professional identity politics orchestrated by titles, coupled with a monopoly on clinical-psychotherapeutic knowledge under the auspices of the controlled act, will not protect the public. It will only limit the number of available clinicians in the province. It will also ensure homogeneity in psychotherapeutic practice.

The proliferation of titles is not only confusing but also borders on the absurd. Even seasoned clinicians will struggle to differentiate between a Psychologist and a Psychological Associate as discerned by the College of Psychologists of Ontario. Few understand what differentiates Social Workers, Psychotherapists, Registered Social Worker Psychotherapists, and OCSWSSW Psychotherapists in the OCSWSSW. Nor does the difference between Psychiatrists and Physicians hold clinical water when physicians can perform the controlled act without psychotherapy training and, like psychiatrists, prescribe medications in accordance with the College of Physicians and Surgeons of Ontario (CPSO). The difference between Certified Nurse Psychotherapists (CNP), Registered Nurses (RN), Registered Practical Nurses (RPN), and Nurse Practitioners (NP) are also not obvious to those outside the medical clinic.[15]

Unregulated providers, those who refuse or who are unable to join one of the Colleges, must work without a registered title. This position outside or beyond the nomenclature of the College, the legislation, the regulators, the malpractice insurers, etc., involves occupying a place of Symbolic non-being, a Real (unsymbolizable) schism in the socio-legal edifice. Like Antigone (who Lacan associates with the psychoanalytic act), the unregulated provider exists in unauthorized territory. They work in a position of legal limbo. As such, they may be disproportionately subject to disciplinary investigation and allegations that they have committed, or are committing, the controlled act without authorization.

Consider Kathryn Walsh of St. Catharines, Ontario, an unregulated provider who was subject to legal action initiated by the College for allegedly "holding herself out as a psychotherapist." Given that Walsh is not a member of a College authorizing her to commit the controlled act, it is the CRPO's position that clients should not be under the impression that she is a psychotherapist. The Application was resolved without a hearing and

Ms. Walsh agreed not to refer to herself as a psychotherapist. According to the Minutes of Settlement for her Superior Court hearing, she agreed to provide the CRPO with a photograph of her business directory, a template of an invoice/receipt issued to clients; confirmation that she had destroyed written materials in which she refers to herself as a psychotherapist; and that the College may "contact her or visit her office to verify whether she is in compliance with the Psychotherapy Act, RHPA and these Minutes of Settlement." Additionally, Walsh had to pay the CRPO $500 to cover the costs of the Application to the Superior Court of Justice.

If the College is, in fact, acting out and caught up in a negative transferential relation to its members and non-members alike, we may better understand the persecution of those using unlawful titles as a reiterative enactment. Like young children, the CRPO makes a scene. Acting out demonstrates that something in the order of signifiers, in this case, titles and psychotherapeutic acts, has been misunderstood. The actions taken against non-members literalizes an error in a performative way. As such, these test-cases are used to make a signifying point. Let us remember that acting out is, in colloquial terms, called "making a scene." The actor is calling upon the audience to acknowledge something that has been missed. We are not really dealing with public protection, but with a problem operating at the level of titles, and thus signification. My point is that the College's enactments are less about the unlawful use of titles than with what has yet to be interpreted.

Let me consider an older psychoanalytic case to make my point. There was a case analyzed by Austrian psychoanalyst Ernst Kris (1900–1957) involving a man who, after his psychoanalytic session, goes off in search of fresh brains to eat. The client worries that he has plagiarized scholarly works. He worries without an external legal agent (an actual other) having made an accusation. The man cannot even say with any degree of certainty that he read the works he accuses himself of having plagiarized. Lacan did not treat this man but referred to the case in *Seminar III*. Lacan ultimately critiques Kris for having misunderstood the man and for adopting an ego-psychological approach to analytic work. But most relevant for our purposes is the assessment Lacan makes about the role of Symbolic ownership for the "Fresh Brains Man" (as he comes to be called). As Hewitson points out, "in the symbolic there is no property, no ownership" (*LacanOnline.com*). In other words, ideas cannot be owned. Like psychotherapy and, ultimately, psychoanalysis, knowledge and signifiers cannot be owned, let alone controlled. It is true, we may search for, find, and punish those who plagiarize the published works of others along with those who commit unlawful psychotherapeutic acts, use the wrong title, and so forth, but ideas, as many copyright lawyers would agree, exist in the public realm.

As with Lacan's critique of the Fresh Brains Man case, the focus upon titles and controlled acts misses the significatory point as it relates to the Controlled Act of Psychotherapy as well. In other words, the CRPO misses the Thing of greatest significance to psychoanalysis and, ultimately, to the public. The administrative actors of the College are, like the Fresh Brains Man, worried about credentials, accreditation, identity, ownership, and copyright. They do not seem to understand that the signifier slides and that authenticity, at the level of professional identity, cannot be ratified. We owe Symbolic debts to others, including those unregulated providers who have devoted their lives to mental health service provision. It is better to acknowledge a debt to the Other than to keep others out by establishing a professional-territorial monopoly.

The College of psychotherapy, like any professional consortium, restricts its members. It is not easy to qualify for registration, and many applicants are denied. Employees of the College, like the man with fresh brains (who searches for the stolen idea-object in texts authored by Others), compulsively check the credentials, citations (advertisements), prefixes, and titles of registered and non-registered members. There is, in the operations of the College, a demand for recognition. A demand for recognition operates on the level of the Symbolic. The Symbolic is like an inheritance; it is something we are bequeathed. A truly original act does not occur through regulations or by compulsively checking to see if one's work is authentic (as the Fresh Brains Man does). It occurs at the level of desire. The actual brains of concern to the Kris case matter less to Lacan than the desire to search for and to find them. Thus, the Lacanian analyst is obliged to intervene at the level of desire, not at the level of the Symbolic (the law).

The search for plagiarists, like the search for those who are in violation of the controlled act, does not end because it is, in Lacanian terms, a repetition. Like all repetitions, the scene must be acted out again. The psychoanalytic objective, for the Fresh Brains Man, is to dispel the idea that "something can only have a value if it belongs to someone else" (Leader 56). Value comes only from the Other in the phantasy of this man. My supposition is that the College is plagued by a similar phantasy but, unlike the Fresh Brains Man, the institution (functioning as agent) is not looking for fresh psychoanalytic acts. As Hewitson points out, for the clinical case,

> it is not the brains in a restaurant that interest the Fresh Brains Man but those being discussed in his analysis – the realm of ideas and the question of who has ownership of them, a question which, given the context of a family history in which he, his father and his grandfather are all academics, is especially pertinent to him.
>
> (LacanOnline.com)

The object, fresh brains, causes the desire of the analysand. It is what brings him, as Hewitson explains, into psychoanalysis. As such, the consumption of ideas (represented by the ingestion of fresh brains in the restaurant) are not actual citational objects but, rather, object causes of desire (*object a*) that propel analysis. There is, in other words, something left unsignified that bothers the man in search of fresh brains.

The College does not really care about the analysis of fresh brains so much as it cares care about the regulation of titles, compliance, and control. It is acting out and, in so doing, refusing to let the psychotherapist sit in the place of lack, in a position of unknowability. In *Seminar XVI*, Lacan says in relation to the analyst (as object cause of desire), that

> in a word, in analysis, the uninterpretable, is the presence of the analyst, and that is why to interpret him as has been seen, as has even been printed, is properly to open the door to what is called this place, namely, acting out.
>
> (qtd. in Hewitson *LacanOnline.com*)

In the legalese of the College, there is no exit. The act is bound to legal repetition. There can be no jumping off the legal stage, so to speak. This is the difference, as Hewitson notes, between "staging a scene on one hand, [and] leaving the scene on the other."

The Psychoanalytic Act

The psychoanalytic act, unlike the controlled act, requires the actor, as analysand, to take leave or, shall we say in Lacanese, a pass. Acting out is to be distinguished from what Lacan calls a passage to the act (*passage à l'acte*).[16] Acting out is always to and for the Other. The subject wants the Other's desire and recognition but fails, in the repetitive loop, to understand that the Other as such does not exist and cannot remedy a lack in being inaugurated by a significatory cut. The traversal of the fundamental fantasy involves an encounter with the Other's desire, a subjective battle on a phantasmatic stage that reveals a lack in being. An internal schism, an impasse, or subjective split is metabolized by the subject-analysand when the fantasy is crossed. A subjective severance is enabled by the act. In other words, the subject is no longer tethered to the Other in a symptomatic way.

The Lacanian act is something the analyst enables, but the act is undertaken by the analysand (albeit unconsciously). The act is authorized by the subject, and they take responsibility for it. As such, it is original and particular to the subject. Following the psychoanalytic act, the subject is forever changed. The act precedes the law and the Symbolic. As such, new signifiers come into being in the afterward. Another way to think about the psychoanalytic act is to suggest that it operates on the Symbolic by taking leave from the Other in a purely subjective way. The act enables the subject to assume a position in relation to the Other's lack. In orchestrating a new subjective position (what Calum Neill calls "a new norm"), the analysand assumes "responsibility in the field of the

Other" (Neill 6). Should the analyst attempt to control or commit the act on behalf of the analysand, they cease to be an analyst. Analysts are, in the Lacanian formulation, *presumed* to know. But they do not know and must become inconsequential to the analysand over the course of analysis.[17]

The psychoanalytic act is a subjective assumption that alters the subject. It enables the subject to dissolve the transference and marks the end of analysis. Unlike acting out, the passage to the act lacks a performative appeal to the Other. The analysand authorizes themselves to act in conformity with their desire, not the law. As such, the act does not have a guarantor. No legislator or actuary will underwrite the act. It occurs at or beyond a Symbolic limit. It is Real and governed by the law of desire. In his discussion of the Lacanian act and Antigone (the Sophocles heroine who remains true to her desire), Neill explains that the "act in this sense should be understood to be coterminous with the emergence of desire; the act is desire made manifest" (2).

Unlike the controlled act that operates in the Symbolic (akin to Antigone's uncle, King Creon's "No!"), the psychoanalytic act occurs in the register beyond signification. It is, thus, a negative act. The subject says "no." But this is no ordinary "no"; it is a refusal of the Symbolic order at a critical juncture in time (to be distinguished from a psychosis involving an ongoing Symbolic foreclosure).[18] The battle is waged at the level of the signifier, not at the level of the body. "The act, therefore, is in the 'no!' – the moment of absolute negativity – because in an act that is successful because it misfires and reinscribes (i.e. fails and recreates) the Symbolic" (Matheou 338). In Lacanian terms, the act must fail (or misfire) if it is to generate something new. It is this failure, the accident, that paradoxically enables a passage to the act.

But the psychoanalytic act need not be in opposition to the law. The Lacanian act reconfigures the Symbolic structure as experienced by the analysand, which is not the same as saying that the psychoanalytic act opposes the law. The significatory shift particular to the subject is a new calculus the law has yet to compute. As Neill explains, the act does not have to be illegal or dangerously transgressive. Referring to an ethics of the act, Neill explains that the act involves a

> subjective response in the face of the system. This does not then mean, however, that the space of ethics is contra the law or system in the base sense of being against the letter of the law, in which case it would necessarily be determined by the law or system. It is rather that the ethical, in being that which the law cannot contain, is beyond or outside the law or system . . . the ethical [can]not be reduced to the law, but neither can it be reduced to an aberration of the law.
>
> (15)

By this, Neill means to say that the good of the psychoanalytic act cannot be judged by the law. It is precisely that which has no bearing or precedent in the law. Just like King Creon could not understand Antigone's steadfast desire to bury her brother in Theban soil, the law cannot discern the singularity of the psychoanalytic act.

To put this another way, the law is not equal to the psychoanalytic act as Lacan understood it. No disciplinary tribunal will uncover a breach in the law equal to what a psychoanalyst enables when working with a client who, in their own time and way, acts psychoanalytically, that is, without being subject to the demand of the Other. The Lacanian act is about a refusal to compromise on one's desire, a refusal to cede ground to the Other (as Symbolic stand-in).

Conclusion

The discourse of the public good provides a justification for a psychotherapy act that mitigates against the psychoanalytic cure as Lacan understood it. Lacanian psychoanalysis, and indeed all psychodynamic interventions, are at risk when the subject of the unconscious is replaced by the subject of disorders. The subject of disorders and impairments, objective assessments, and ready-made psychotherapeutic treatment protocols of interest to the College is at odds with the subject of the unconscious that is internally divided by language. What distinguishes Lacanian psychoanalysis from the Controlled Act of Psychotherapy is a commitment to a particular (subjective) ethics, an ethic of desire, irreducible to the subject of psychological assessment. The master's signifiers, the rules of law, regulation, and control cease to operate for the subject when the client-analysand commits the psychoanalytic act.

The psychoanalytic act cannot be reconciled with the discourse of the College or the legislation authorizing it. There is something lost when questions relating to desire and unconscious processes are replaced by assessment tools predicated upon historically contingent psychological and psychiatric norms. Psychoanalytic acts are foreclosed when the clinician's response is determined by a "pre-given system of knowledge" (Neill 8). There is, in the College's entry-to-practice requirements, a refusal to acknowledge a lack or gap in knowing and acting. The presumption to know is dangerous, especially when working psychotherapeutically with clients. The legislation imposes a method of clinical psychotherapeutic practice that disregards the analytic value of not-knowing. It is about professional control, liability, accountability, transparency, measurement, outcomes, adjustment, diagnosis, and best professional practice at odds with the psychoanalytic cure. Over a century of psychoanalytic research, teaching, and clinical practice, Lacanian and otherwise, is being replaced by a legal-judicial approach to client care more amenable to governments and insurance companies than to people.

Notes

1 I use Other (with a capital "O") to refer to the alterity of language, the law, and the Symbolic. I will use other (with a lower case "o") to refer to ego-based projections of others (relevant to the imaginary register), as opposed to actual people.

2 The College is run by a council comprised of six to nine members elected by psychotherapists registered by the College and eight persons appointed by the Lieutenant Governor. Two of the elected members are chosen to be president and vice-president. As written on the CRPO website, their mandate is to regulate its members with respect to the "professional, legal and ethical requirements governing their practice [as psychotherapists]."

3 The RHPA was amended in 2007 to include psychotherapy as a controlled act.

4 Subsection 11 makes CRPO regulations governing psychotherapeutic practice subject to Ministerial review and approval by the Lieutenant Governor in Council. The powers of the Minister include the right to review the council's activities, to require the council to provide reports and information upon request and to make, amend, or revoke a regulation under the act including "anything that, in the opinion of the Minister, is necessary or advisable to carry out the intent of this [RHPA] Act" (2007, c. 10, Sched. R, s. 12 (5)).

5 New Brunswick and Nova Scotia regulate titles affiliated with therapy and counselling. In 2018 Alberta passed legislation regulating counselling, and a College of Counselling Therapy of Alberta (CCTA) will oversee the relevant mental health and addictions services. But no existing regulation compares to the Controlled Act of Psychotherapy.

6 According to "The Therapeutic Relationship as the Cornerstone of the Controlled Act of Psychotherapy" (2017) (a document prepared for the Minister by the Health Professions Regulatory Advisory Council), CPSO is quoted as follows: "The definition of psychotherapy set out in the legislation is technically inaccurate and does not align with the medical model for psychotherapeutic treatment and therefore the clarification document is also problematic. Most serious disorders as defined in the document would not be treated with psychotherapy, either as primary or adjunct treatment. . . . Most patients/clients who currently receive psychotherapy would not be included under this definition and therefore the "risk of harm" which is inherent in all of the controlled acts would not apply to them even though there are risks of harm for these individuals who are receiving psychotherapy" (16).

7 OPSEU explains that the Act "could pose challenges for many OPSEU members who work as addiction counsellors, rape crisis workers, supportive housing workers, child and youth workers, and in other occupations" (https://opseu.org/news/change-to-psychotherapy-act-could-pose-challenges-for-counsellors-others/16980/).

8 OPSEU notes that since 2015, when the CRPO became operational, the lack of clarity relating to the controlled act has "contributed to fewer psychotherapy services being available to the public" (https://opseu.org/news/change-to-psychotherapy-act-could-pose-challenges-for-counsellors-others/16980/). Particularly alarming is the elimination of jobs and provisions allocated for community mental health support.

9 It is worth noting that the College initially rejected applicants for registration who used single-session therapy (SST) hours to count toward the clinical hours required for registration until they were forced through a successful legal appeal in 2019 to recognize SST as psychotherapy. The College did not believe that a single session was equal to a therapeutic relationship that "evolve[s] over time" (Young and Jebreen, 35).

10 In *Practice Guidelines for Performing the Controlled Act of Psychotherapy*, the Ontario College of Social Workers and Social Service Workers (OCSWSSW) wrote about the lack of clarity between psychotherapy services and counselling services. They openly acknowledge that the distinction between the two are "challenging in practice." They also write that, "ultimately, it is anticipated that the courts and College discipline committees will provide guidance on what is or is not included within the Controlled Act of Psychotherapy" (5).
11 The Ministry of Health and Long Term Care (MOHLTC) instructed the College to further define and refine the Act. The CRPO produced a YouTube video, a Self Assessment Tool, and other documents available on their website to clarify the status of the controlled act.
12 A provider may also join the Ontario College of Social Workers and Social Services Workers (OCSWSSW), which would enable them to commit the Controlled Act of Psychotherapy, a College not under the jurisdiction of the RHPA.
13 See www.stoppsychotherapytakeover.ca/ and www.eenetconnect.ca/topic/the-uncontrolled-act-of-psychotherapy.
14 For example, the founder and at least one instructor of the three-year psychoanalytic psychotherapy training program at the Toronto Institute for Contemporary Psychotherapy (TICP) maintain that politics are not relevant to psychotherapy.
15 It should be noted that psychotherapy titles now exceed the bounds of the clinic and the hospital. They are appearing in the arts, areas I would have thought protected from legislative control. Consider, for example, that Amy Clements-Cortés of Wilfred Laurier University, a music scholar, establishes a difference between "music psychotherapy" and "music therapy". Music psychotherapists allegedly use the medical model of psychotherapy authorized by the College, while music therapists do not.
16 See Lacan, Jacques. *The Seminar of Jacques Lacan: Book X, Anxiety 1962–1963* for a discussion of the passage to the act.
17 In *Seminar X*, Lacan writes that the analysand is reduced to *objet a* when they make the passage to the act. They are, in other words, identified with the *a*.
18 Lacan calls this *aphanisis*.

Works Cited

Breuer, Joseph, Sigmund Freud. *Studies on Hysteria*. 1985. Basic Books, 2000.

Clements-Cortés, Amy. "Music Therapy Implications: The College of Registered Psychotherapists of Ontario." *Canadian Music Educator*, vol. 58, no. 1, 2016, pp. 39–41.

Eliany, Geneviève. "Psychotherapy Takeover Fears III: Call for Feedback. Discussion Paper." *elianylaw.ca*. Accessed 16 June 2021, buckleyandco.ca/documents/CRPOsurvey.pdf.

Freud, Sigmund. *Civilization and Its Discontents*, edited by James Strachey. 1930. W.W. Norton & Company, 2010.

Freud, Sigmund. "Totem and Taboo." *The Standard Edition of the Complete Psychological Works of Sigmund Freud, Volume XIII (1913–1914): Totem and Taboo and Other Works*. Hogarth Press, 1955, pp. 1–162.

Health Professions Regulatory Advisory Council. *Regulation of Health Professions in Ontario: New Directions*. Province of Ontario, 2006.

Hewitson, Owen. "What Does Lacan Say About . . . Acting Out?" *LacanOnline.com*. Accessed 16 June 2021, www.lacanonline.com/2010/12/what-does-lacan-say-about-acting-out/.

Kristeva, Julia. *New Maladies of the Soul*. Columbia University Press, 1995.

Lacan, Jacques. *The Seminar of Jacques Lacan: Book I, Freud's Papers on Technique 1953–1954*, edited by Jacques-Alain Miller. Translated by John Forrester. W.W. Norton & Company, 1991.

Lacan, Jacques. *The Seminar of Jacques Lacan: Book III, The Psychoses 1955–1956*, edited by Jacques-Alain Miller. Translated by Russell Grigg, W.W. Norton & Company, 1993.

Lacan, Jacques. *The Seminar of Jacques Lacan: Book V, The Formations of the Unconscious 1957–1958*, edited by Jacques-Alain Miller. Translated by Russell Grigg. W.W. Norton & Company, 2017.

Lacan, Jacques. *The Seminar of Jacques Lacan: Book VII: The Ethics of Psychoanalysis 1959–1960*, edited by Jacques-Alain Miller. Translated by Dennis Porter. W.W. Norton & Company, 1997.

Lacan, Jacques. *The Seminar of Jacques Lacan: Book X: Anxiety 1962–1963*, edited by Jacques-Alain Miller. Translated by A.R. Price. Polity Press, 2014.

Lacan, Jacques. *The Seminar of Jacques Lacan: Book XV: The Psychoanalytic Act 1967–1968*. Translated by Cormac Gallagher. Karnac, 2002.

Lacan, Jacques. *The Seminar of Jacques Lacan: Book XVI: From the Other to the Other 1968–1969*. Translated by Cormac Gallagher. Karnac, 2002.

Lacan, Jacques. *The Seminar of Jacques Lacan: Book XVIII: On a Discourse That Might Not Be a Semblance 1971*. Translated by Cormac Gallagher. Karnac, 2002.

Leader, Darian. *Promises Lovers Make When It Gets Late*. Faber & Faber, 1997.

Malabou, Catherine. *The New Wounded: From Neurosis to Brain Damage*. Translated by Steven Miller. Fordham University Press, 2012.

Matheou, Louis. "The Act Reconsidered: Actcidental Antigone and the New Wounded." *Psychoanalysis, Culture & Society*, vol. 23, no. 3, 2018, pp. 330–349.

Neill, Calum. "An Idiotic Act: On the Non-Example of Antigone." *The Letter*, vol. 34, 2005, pp. 1–28.

Ontario Superior Court of Justice. "Minutes of Settlement Between College of Registered Psychotherapists and Registered Mental Health Therapists of Ontario and Sandra Fecht." *College of Registered Psychotherapists of Ontario*. Accessed 16 June 2021, www.crpo.ca/wp-content/uploads/2017/11/Sandra-Fecht-1.pdf.

Psychotherapy Act. *Statutes of Ontario, c.10, Schedule R. Ontario*. Legislative Assembly of the Province of Ontario. 2007. *Ontario*. Web. 16 June 2021.

Young, Karen, Joseph Jebreen. "Recognizing Single-Session Therapy as Psychotherapy." *Journal of Systemic Therapies*, vol. 38, no. 4, 2019, pp. 31–44.

Chapter 9

Groups and Communality

A Real Conundrum for the Social World

Eve Watson

Introduction: Functions and Vicissitudes of a Group

Most psychoanalysts are members of a psychoanalytic group and find them to be an invaluable support for what can be an enjoyable but sometimes isolated psychoanalytic clinical practice. The significance of a group affiliation is unique to each member and is usually exemplified in their relation to the group: some members are more active than others, some are inactive, others seek organisational positions in a group. For both Freud and Lacan, the psychoanalytic group was crucial to the work of the transmission of psychoanalysis. For them, it simply wasn't enough for this to be left to individual psychoanalysts, and a collective effort was necessary. Moreover, there were concerns that some might set up their own schools. As we know, some of their closest colleagues did go on to do that.[1] Lacan's colourful history and management of his own psychoanalytic groups is an important aspect of his teaching and was adjudged by him to be elemental to the transmission of psychoanalysis and key to distinguishing his school from the established psychoanalytic institutions of which he was deeply critical. Lacan did not offer a theory of groups but established his school, the École Freudienne de Paris, in 1964, which went through several iterations as he sought to keep it relevant to his aims until he dissolved it in 1980 and shortly thereafter established a new group, the École de la Cause Freudienne. Lacan never stopped interrogating the function, success, and failure of his psychoanalytic group and instituted reforms, invention, and dissolution in an ongoing effort to keep the psychoanalytic group fresh, open-minded, creative, and attentive to the new. He had successes and failures along the way. Both Lacan and Freud offer us much to evaluate groups and "communality."

Groups, as Freud (1921/2001) proposed in "Group Psychology," have an important role in organising the sacrifice of drive-satisfaction or *jouissance* necessary for going beyond narcissistic satisfaction and redirecting it onto social and communal aims. Freud marvelled at the success of the communal realm in providing substitutive satisfaction and a limited pleasure.

DOI: 10.4324/9781003212072-10

Asserting that individual psychology is at the same time social psychology (ibid., 69), the drive for sociability has its origins in the family unit or group. A group as such acts as a container for anxiety, allowing people to unify to pursue agreed upon aims and redirecting individual narcissism onto the group's work, which is typically dominated by a leader/master. In his analysis of group effects, Freud perceives that group membership has certain effects and causes individuals to change due to:

1. the intensification of affects and
2. the diminution of intellectual activity (ibid.).

Simply put, group members are expected to rein in their own views in favour of the group's, and group activity can support the removal of inhibitions, leading to a level of drive satisfaction. The political and social domain is rife with examples from cults to proto-nationalistic groups who often refuse accepted knowledge and are "driven" by the group's affective bond and idealisation of the leader. The intensification of affects, which requires some action, is often managed by directing it at another group or something outside of the group, which can have a binding effect tantamount to a common or shared identity among the group members and, in particular, with the group leader. A Donald Trump rally during the US Presidential election campaign in 2020 offers a paradigmatic exemplar containing all of these elements: the refusal to believe in the accepted knowledge of COVID-19 and distrust of all mainstream news; an unfaltering faith in the leader; and the affective enjoyment of the rally participants was unmistakeable in "lock her up" in reference to Hilary Clinton, in the mass mockery of a disabled reporter, in repeated horde-like attacks on reporters, and the storming of the US Congress building in Washington in January 2021. The basis, Freud writes, of these relationships is love, which "constitute[s] the essence of the group mind" (ibid., 91). Transference love powerfully serves to keep the group together through libidinal ties to the leader and each other, and as we know, this has an idealising aspect. This facilitates a triumphal feeling in allowing the ego to coincide with the ego ideal (ibid., 131), which can be much harder to attain in reality. Ambivalence in the group is typically managed by directing love at the leader and hatred outward at what is perceived to be the cause of discontent. This can go as far as taking on a delusional or mass delirium aspect, as some have reported in the case of Trump supporters who revere him and take a deeply antagonistic approach to those who do not support him (Lewis 2021).

Let us pause for a moment and consider what an ideal is, and specifically its function in an analysis. As Freud noted, idealisation implies overestimating the object and is always a source of tension under the sway of the demands of the super-ego. Ideals are implicated in identification and therefore inevitable, and a psychoanalyst expects to work with them, being the basis of transference love in an analysis. In other words, the analysand idealises the analyst during an analysis. But, as Serge Cottet notes, the analyst does not work to support the analysand's ideals or to ease the tension between ideals and the demands of the super-ego, but rather works to accentuate their radical difference. In doing this, the analyst works from the basis that the analysand's ideals are not the measure of the legitimacy of their desires (Cottet 2012, 127). In order to do this, the analyst takes up a position as not the ideal but rather the object a, the object cause of desire. There is a big gap between them, the ideal and the object a, and this is the basis of tension. A group can be a place onto which this tension is displaced and finds an object. Groups provide a range of desirable and transferential objects in their members, work and activities, aims, and actions to meet this tension.

Furthermore, the analyst does not pursue an ideal of her own with an analysand, including one that is therapeutically curative, and instead leaves it up to the analysand to choose her own path according to the constituent nature of her desire. Indeed, the more the patient seeks to be cured, the more the analyst should look to whether she is augmenting this via her own desire driven by curative ideals. The analyst's cool, privative, even apathetic approach to the elimination of the analysand's symptom and her well-being is possible only with the abandonment of pursing an ideal of cure, and it brings out the analysand's frustration, which re-emphasises the real effects of the prohibition of *jouissance*. It is in managing the satisfactions derived from *jouissance* that a curative effect is achieved by the analysand, not by idealising and identifying with the analyst. For an analyst, a psychoanalytic group can serve as a place for the satisfaction of an identification or ideal, a transposition if you will, of the analyst's ideals from the domain of the clinical room to the communal setting, where they are less likely to interfere with the analyst's neutrality. This can be an important displacement onto the psychoanalytic group and a potentially important outlet for the analyst's satisfaction.

The trouble with this, as Freud notes in his chapter on identification in "Group Psychology," is the ambivalence of identification, as from the beginning the affect of love can just as easily turn to hate (1921/2001, 105). One way a group deals with its internal ambivalence is to direct hatred onto another group and externalise it outside of the group. This takes advantage of the fact that our primary identification that allows us to distinguish between inside and outside is alienating and structures our relationship to the world and knowledge in a paranoic way, leaving us with the suspicion that the outside never stops impinging, even on the self (1949/2006, 77). This is indicated in conspiracy theories such as those promoted by QAnon, which assert that paranoid idea that we are constantly under observation and management by a global cabal of corrupt leaders and QAnon followers who have a special inside knowledge of this and the apocalypse to come (LaFrance 2020).

Importantly, group membership can fulfil a double function of moderating ambivalent affects while also facilitating regression, if we take Freud's assertion that identification is the most primitive emotional tie, precedes object choice, and can easily become a substitute for an object (1921/2001, 107). The fact that others are members of the group is the basis for the perception of mutuality, commonality, and similarity between them (ibid., 107–108) and is the identificatory basis of empathy. The role of identification in empathy is that it provides a substitute pathway by limiting aggressivity towards those the individual has identified with, allowing help to be offered and a clan feeling to develop (ibid., 110). This regression to identification can, however, take on a slavish or extremely devoted hue when the object is too loved and the identification and introjection of the object replaces the ego ideal, thereby diminishing the moral imperatives and conscience of the person. The recent example of Trump supporters exemplifies this: they claim they overlook Trump's unabashedly misogynistic and racist qualities because he is a good businessman and leader (Gabriel 2021), in spite of evidence that he has not been successful in business but instead has manipulated tax schemes and successfully managed mountains of debt.

As this shows, group identification causes time and again the weakening of the intellectual capacity of its individuals, the disinhibition of impulses, and the lifting of moderation, impelling action to work these off. What defines groups is often the actions permitted to work these off and whether the work supports the group or community or is antagonistically directed outward at another group. The role of the group leader can in point of this be understood in relation to uncanny and coercive aspects of group formations and specifically the dreaded primal father who encapsulates the group ideal and takes over the individual ego ideal (Freud 1921/2001, 127). Such a group leader looms large and is a dominating and overwhelming force, without whom group members imagine they would be helpless. This facilitates the idea that it is impossible to live in the world and be outside of some group, whether ethnic, religious, national, racial, and so on. What then of psychoanalytic groups, and do they mirror these qualities that Freud noted about groups generally? Have psychoanalytic groups figured out how to support individuals in communality?

Freud and the Invention of a Psychoanalytic Group

The first psychoanalytic group was Freud's Wednesday night reading group in Freud's residence, which was, according to Peter Gay, formed "with the declared intention of learning, practicing, and disseminating psychoanalysis" (Gay 1998, 173). Its significance was such that there was, according to Gay, an atmosphere of the foundation of a religion in the room. It was always thus going to be more than a reading group, and after several years, in 1908 the Vienna Society was formed as Freud's writing became more known, and it began to collect a library. Subsequently, the International Psychoanalytic Association (IPA) was founded in 1910 after the first international psychoanalytic congress in Salzburg in 1909. In its founding, by bringing together the various local branches in places such as Berlin, Budapest, Zurich, Vienna, and the USA, Freud hoped to create a movement and bring analysts together in a closer bond, given the increasing success and recognition of psychoanalysis. There had been a growing problem of dissension among valued adherents, such as Jung, and with the founding the IPA, Freud hoped to unify these diffuse elements. His paper at the second International Congress in 1910 was on "The Future Prospects of Psycho-Analytic Therapy," which spoke to these themes and his wish that psychoanalysis would extend well beyond its Viennese origins (Freud 1910/2001). But the IPA's beginning was fraught with discontent and disagreement, mainly due to Sandor Ferenczi's imperiousness and disagreement over procedural matters. Added to this, the appointment by Freud of Carl Jung as the first president of the IPA in 1910 did not go over well, as Jung's qualities were more rebellious and son-like than father-like, as one would expect in a leader (Jones 1961, 329).

Prior to the establishment of the IPA, Freud made an interesting proposal at one of the Vienna Society's Wednesday evenings in 1908. He proposed the dissolution of their Wednesday night group and the resignations of members who should re-join each year. He explained this would take account of inevitable changes in the relationships between members that could cause them to feel obliged to remain as members lest their action of resigning be taken as unfriendly. This process, Freud explained, has "the purpose of re-establishing the personal freedom of each individual and of making it possible for him to stay apart from the Society without in any way disturbing his relations with the rest of us" (Jones 1961, 314). This lasted only until 1910 but was retained by Swiss and British societies in order to restrict membership to serious students of psychoanalysis.

This can be considered as a valuable mode in which group members resubmit their group membership in a formal way each year and governing committees and leadership change often; this is how a group allows for the desire of individual members to be expressed about being members of the group. As Gay notes, a psychoanalytic group is not easy to maintain, as sparks of hostility are inevitable with sensitive individuals sometimes working together; the provocative subject matter of psychoanalytic enquiry can touch on "some of the most heavily guarded spots of the human psyche," which takes a toll and can generate "a pervasive irritability" among the members and in their interactions with each other (Gay 1998, 177). There is thus much to be said of the importance for groups of renewing, re-forming, and changing aspects of its structures in order to counter the tendency of groups towards stagnation, infighting, and splitting.

We can also ask what it means to transform the private psychoanalytic treatment of an individual into public events and writings via a group mechanism. Extending links to a wider audience is an important way for psychoanalysis to develop and grow, but the disparity between the private world of the individual's sexuality, phantasies, symptoms, and dreams and that of the public and political dimension of the movement of psychoanalysis is significant and unbridgeable. Added to this is the offensive nature of what psychoanalysis has to say to rationality-minded and moralistic sensibilities. Coming to recognise this, Adam Philips notes that unlike followers such as Wilhelm Reich and Paul Federn, Freud became less interested in the political dimension of his work and writing. As a result of the varied reactions of those in his group, which reminded him of what he had omitted or repressed in his writing and elaborations, he became more interested in the therapeutic efficacy of his theories and concepts (Philips 2014, 129). Freud's writing and public face had initially served to bring authority to the psychoanalytic cause and was the basis of his early writing, but with the development of the small, dynamic, and mixed Vienna Society group into what became the IPA, Freud's writing became increasingly less technical and more accessible to the interested reader (Phillips, 133).

Freud demonstrated the immutable sociability of individuals who, even in a psychoanalytic group, commune with each other, read each other's minds, and take pleasure in these activities, what Lacan would call *jouissance*. This is the province of a psychoanalytic group no less than any other, and how these activities, some imaginary, some symbolic, and some real, are recognised and accommodated determines the group. Philips notes that as time went on it became increasingly clear to Freud and others that psychoanalysis as a profession became more obsessed with enforcing its own rules of theory and practice than in considering what the rules were for (Phillips, 147–148). In a Jewish way, "desire for the law would trump all other desires," as Phillips notes (ibid.) The development of strict didactic mechanisms of training and the formalisation of study by psychoanalytic institutions was a kind of acculturation of psychoanalysis that Foucault would rightfully describe as having become embedded in strategies of knowledge and power (Foucault 1990, 73). Freud answered this by writing increasingly to a non-technical audience and seeking to spread the work of psychoanalysis beyond its institutions.

Lacan and Group Psychology

In 1964, Lacan founded his school, the École Freudians de Paris, and embarked on a very different path to that of established and powerful French psychoanalytic institutions. He explains his actions and ethical imperative:

> That is why it is not sufficient for us for the moment, here, simply to ground the status of the analyst, in a way, in an arbitrary fashion

> prefigured by our categories; it is a matter of seeing whether our categories are not those which allow us precisely to construct the map, to understand what is involved in one or other theoretical tendency in the analytic milieu, in the community of analysts, with this position which in each analyst – and quite naturally not simply in an isolated fashion but in the measure of the experience that he has had of it, namely his formative experience – of what in each analyst can be located in terms of a desire that is an essential reference for him.
>
> (Lacan, 1964–65, Session: 17 March 1965, 163)

Lacan's approach to the transmission of psychoanalysis and the organising of psychoanalysts into a group was driven not by the need for consensus but rather for as open-minded an approach to training as possible (Hofstein, 167). Lacan had already remarked in the previous decade that Freud's "Group Psychology," which was written ten years after the IPA was established, allowed him to keenly observe group dynamics and led him to discover the importance of identification with the group ego ideal. The group ego ideal is, according to Lacan, a "phenomenon of infatuation" and imaginary identification and proposes, "the mirage of which is borne by the personality of the leader. A sensational discovery which slightly anticipated the fascistic organisations that rendered it obvious" (1956/2006, 397). This is how groups are undemocratic and, as "democracies of masters," are modelled on the democracy of Antiquity (ibid.) with members whose forms are facsimiles. They are "copies whereby the one becomes plural" (ibid., 398). Collective identification, Lacan continues, is modelled on an ideal of "sufficiency" that does not encourage speech but, on the contrary, constrains it so that group effects are uniformly maintained (ibid., 400). This is a communing in which narcissistic identification, jealousy, and acrimony find fertile soil. What underpins this is "knowledge in a pathetic form" in which people "commune without communicating" and where hatred breeds in a knowledge vacuum (ibid.) This is knowledge spawned by de-intellectualisation, and it is affectively loaded. In a comment that gives pause for thought, Lacan asserts that "ideals are society's slaves" (ibid., 705). While this is a criticism directed at psychology, it points to how any group can end up being enslaved to social ideals once ideals are given free rein in a group. Those ideals inevitably end up supporting norms and dominant ideological trends such as the market, consumption, and gender ideals; since 9/11, Islamophobia; and during the COVID-19 pandemic, anti-Asian bias.

So why bother with a group, then, when culture, as only Lacan could put it, "discharges us from the function of thinking" (Lacan 1967–68/2008, 67) and, in extension, refers to groups and Freud's observation of the diminution of intellectual work by group membership and activities? How thus then to create and maintain a psychoanalytic society, one that can withstand the idealising and de-intellectualising tendencies of the communal and remain open to new knowledge and invention of its analyst members? On the one hand, a group needs a leader, and there all kinds of leaders: some are temperate, some perverse, some overbearing, others masterful and narcissistic. Good or bad, what is crucial is how any group manages the toxic and disruptive effect of transferential investment and imaginary projections on to the figure of a group leader and, in so doing, make them a master. Both Freud and Lacan recognised therein lay trouble. Freud quietly withdrew from the burgeoning association (IPA) he had instituted, although his voice remained powerfully active. Later, Lacan (1980) decried those who called themselves "Lacanians," preferring to call himself a Freudian in what was a criticism of the idealising transference to him and his teaching.

De-Emphasising Ideals in Group Dynamics

> That is why transference is a relationship that is essentially tied to time and its handling. But what is the being that responds to us, operating in the field of speech and language, from shy of the cave's entrance? I would go so far as to embody it in the form of the very walls of the cave that would (like to) live or rather come alive with palpitations whose living movement must be grasped now – that is, now that I have articulated the function and field of speech and language in their conditioning
>
> (Lacan 1964/2006, 716)

Transference undoubtedly operates in groups and institutions as well as in the clinic. It also has a political dimension when used as a mode of power. As Andrew Lewis notes, the "intrinsic relationship" between politics and transference reminds us that the analyst's position is not neutral, requiring an act that ultimately can be judged only at an ethical level (Lewis 2000, 138–139). As for the psychoanalytic act, Moustapha Safouan reminds us that the act (interpretation, intervention, silence, cut, etc.) is sustained by the analyst's desire, as is his or her bond among analysts in the transference to the work that maintains analysis as necessary to permanent formation (Safouan 2003, 2). Safouan explains that formation, as in the formation of the analyst, emerges as an effect of the formations of the unconscious in concert with analytic listening, and the analyst's desire is a consequence of an analysis, not the cause of one (ibid., 7). Formation, as we know, includes personal analysis, supervision, teaching, presenting of clinical cases, attending seminars, and writing. This is sustained in the work of supporting the transmission of new knowledge and not the already known, pre-established knowledge, as well as considerations of analysts' inventions that are presented to the group or perhaps a sub-section of the group. In this sense, a group is comprised of disparate ones and singular voices that, through a desire to work with the unconscious, dislodge master signifiers, do not pander to ideals of imaginary unity, and leave little room for the domination of imaginary defences.

This is subverted by the "working dimension" of the transference in which institutions and groups forget or ignore that clinical concepts of psychoanalysis are applicable to its institutional structure, which Lacan clearly accepted (Lewis 2000, 141), and when transference is deployed in service of power and political ends. In groups, this is revealed in cronyism and nepotism and functions as a corrupt toxic element that a group deals with by projecting it outward onto others and other groups, or by directing it inward onto the chosen few. This is not a discourse oriented by lack-in-being but is a discourse of semblance offering a fertile terrain for affect and *jouissance* to dominate. *Jouissance* enjoys and will always come back for more. We are back to the problem of what to do with drive affects and *jouissance* at a social level.

As an alternative to the imaginary attributes of groups marked by tendencies to de-intellectualisation and the exacerbation of affects in the field of their relations, Lacan offers an interpretation of Plato's Allegory of the Cave in "The Position of the Unconscious," presented in 1960 but re-written in 1964, from which the quote at the beginning of this section is taken. Here Lacan explores the division of the subject that is linked by him not only to a point outside the cave but to the very walls of the cave itself, which we can designate as the Other. The subject therefore coincides with an edge in relation to the Other that is the source of the subject's division, separation, and castration. But it is through the Other that the subject comes closer to what she has lost and what causes her desire, and also closer to the drive insofar as the body's openings have been thought about and touched by speech. As the Other, the analyst functions as the object that causes desire and provokes the drive through the transference, forcing an enactment with the missed encounter with the analysand's being or being-ness, in order to create something new. This is a unique way of capturing the wager of analysis, and the analyst must not identify with the know-it-all who returns to the cave with his boon of knowledge and pronounces it to the uninterested audience.

> Now, as we know, transference brings with it the best and worst, and when it takes hold on the scale of a group, not to mention a vast group, it becomes indissoluble.
>
> (Safouan 2000, 119)

In the group context, work must be undertaken so that members are not the enchained slaves ensnared in ideology and culture and the group mindset. Groups can take various steps to vitiate against this. One mode is through the elevation of difference into an ethical principle. This is an outcome of the analyst's desire for pure difference, and the uniqueness of subjective desire reminds that the analyst is also an analysand. This takes into account that "there is a real at stake in formation of the psychoanalyst" (Lacan 1967, 3), a fundamental gap, an agalma that undermines the phantasy of inter-subjectivity in which one subject communes directly with another. This is knowledge that contains a hole that cannot be filled with didactic knowledge but is supported by the object cause of desire in its singularity for each group member. Taking this into account means that "the inessentiality of the subject supposed to know is unveiled" (ibid., 13), and each member must find their own symptomatic solution. This is antagonistic to the appeal of the imaginary aspects of unity.

The problem is that transference can cause members to remain in slave-like relations to others who occupy a master position and are supposed to contain knowledge. Instead, a transference to work rooted in lack in being and the empty place of desire allows group members to act in support of their own desire, as distinct to acting in support of the authority of the institution or certain institutional members. What matters is how the group deals with this. As Lewis puts it, "the institution itself must incarnate a politics of the lack-in-being, the empty cause, so as to enable an analytic discourse to handle the transference of its members" (Lewis 2000, 149). I explore next various dynamic, topological, and economic ways in which a psychoanalytic group can do this.

Group coherence is important for group members as it offers a sense of being part of a group and is an effort dedicated to the transmission of psychanalysis. This phrasing is deliberate. Being a "part" of a group points to a group's composition of different parts. One problem is that groups tend to eliminate differences between members, and idealising transferences support this process of producing sameness. This is supported by a hunger for love, the lure of narcissistic mirage, defensiveness, and affective disinhibition. That is not to say that broad agreement and shared aims and values among group members aren't vital, but, if pursued at the cost of an ethics of difference, a group is destined to aggression and eventual splitting.

Lacan bleakly warns that a group defined by imaginary identifications seeks an ideal Father and in promoting "co-existence" as distinct to an ethic of difference can easily slip from humanism to terror with segregation inevitable. This is ultimately "what the term concentration camp renders speakable" (Lacan 1967, 17). Maintaining a group based on the singularity of the lack-in-being of group members is a challenge for any group. If we are to take Lacan at his word and action, maintaining an ethic of difference requires experimentation, constant review, and sometimes even the dissolution of the group in order to start afresh. To consider how groups can be hospitable to alterity and informed by an ethic of difference, I will consider various approaches in light of Freud's triad of categories of the psyche: dynamic, topological, economic (Freud 1915/2001).

A Dynamic, Topological, and Economic Approach to a Group and Communality

A topological approach to the psychoanalytic group emphasises the importance of a group's work taking place in various places at once. First, the work is spread across different locales within the group, such as reading groups or cartels, teaching work, organisational work, writing, and public seminars. A horizontal rather than vertical organisation is one oriented to allowing analysts to find each of those who will support them in a psychoanalytic position, which is the occupation of a hole, of a place not already designated and known. A topological approach also means the group understands it does not work in a vacuum but can function as a place where analysts can direct their attention in a social way to concepts, techniques, and matters of practice on different levels. An emphasis on rigour and attention to psychoanalytic concepts, clinic, and ethics meets with the demands of the group super-ego, and the strength or imperative of this will likely depend on the approach of the group leaders. The work of the group in producing knowledge will be registered across different psychical locales. There are unconscious as well as conscious effects in producing knowledge that will be unique for each member. In other words, the effects of producing knowledge cannot be known or guaranteed in advance for the individual members and the group but are a combination of a dynamic process of interaction between different psychical agencies, some transposed to the group, some working away individually for each group member.

A dynamic approach is premised on whether a group is willing to assess its work and history and what it "allows" into its work, thought, and productions. A dynamically driven group understands that repression is part and parcel of a working group and anxiety is its accompaniment. To moderate this, having new voices and people from outside the group work with the group is important, including voices that diverge from a group's stated or known approach in order for there to be opportunities to reconsider known knowledge. Within the group, are there mechanisms for new and recent members to participate and bring fresh perspectives to it? A horizontal rather than a hierarchical or vertical approach offers opportunities for fresh metonymising and metaphorising (the combinatory of the signifier) within the group and can punctuate the reproduction of old symptoms. New symptoms function by dynamising a group and are indicative of a group that is more open than closed and prone to repetition of old problems and difficulties. This also can limit the tendencies towards idealisation of established members and the infinite promise of revelation of the university discourse. As Safouan notes, a multi-voiced teaching can distribute these transferential investments and "organise a plural transferential terrain around a common cause" (Safouan 2003, 3). This is a kind of dilution of the transference to the master by way of a distribution to working ventures within the group in support of the group's aims.

An economic approach to the group and communal field is premised on how a group manages its libidinal drive affects or *jouissances*, which is perhaps its biggest challenge. As Lewis notes, the singularity of each *jouissance* cannot be a basis of the group (Lewis 2000, 149). As Freud set out, it is work that does this, and his emphasis was on the psychoanalytic act as opposed to acting out the drive and its *jouissance*. Sublimation is one mode of satisfying the drive, and it is economically advantageous at the level of *jouissance* as it avoids repression. As only Lacan could put it, "for the moment, I am not fucking, I am talking to you! Well I can have exactly the same satisfaction as if as if I were fucking, that's what it means" (Lacan, 1964/2004, 165–166). This is a sublimation or deferment of *jouissance* and a focus instead on the network or combinatory of signifier, which is desire. How does a group organise the deferment of *jouissance* at a collective level such that its members go to work? It can be directed to textual work that is oriented to working knowledge obtained by exposing master signifiers and preserving the desire of the analyst and cause as an empty place, so that the analyst is not a slave to the analytic cause. This is a more open, democratic way of working. This is not easy to do because empty cause is embodied in the semblances of authority, and demands made upon the group by its members point to *jouissances* there in each.

Concluding Thoughts

The field of human relations is rife with dialectics of misrecognition, negation, and narcissistic alienation that can easily blight groups and support discourses oriented by a narcissism of small differences. This underlies infighting and disputes with other, often remarkably similar groups. More widely, these emerge socio-culturally in forms identifiable as misogyny, hatred, and racism. To be a practitioner of the symbolic function is to make room for the truth of unconscious desire, which may not equate to interpretations according to norms or ideological models. Taking the Other into account and the subject as divided requires repositioning truth at the heart of social relations, but it can be a painful truth that spotlights human frailty and limitation, as desire is also rooted in loss and frustration. This nonetheless is the analytic discourse, and it founds a social bond in which analysts are responsible for their own work, which is impelled by their desire.

It is nonetheless extraordinarily difficult to maintain a social bond founded on the singularity of desire and the oneness of *jouissance* from the effects of masterising tendencies. Elitism can be impossible to prevent in a group with an unchanging hierarchy, and Lacan discerned his own school had become too "Lacanian" and invested in the "whole" rather than the sum of its parts. In what must have been a painful decision, in 1980 he took the step of dissolving it. He had discerned that his own influence had become too powerful and that the group's failure to adhere to its own aims was in part due to his influence. Thus, Lacan's own group, founded to oppose the elitism of institutionalised psychoanalysis and its "standardised" methods of training, had itself become mired in ideological and political impasse. Lacan didn't just dissolve the École in 1980; in his letter of dissolution, he wrote of returning to the Other (discernible in his statement "I persevere") from whence his radical movement sprung. As Hofstein puts it, for Lacan the group had become "more Lacanian than Lacan" (2010, 172), just as Freud, in his quiet withdrawal and emphasis on technique in his later work, arrived at a similar perspective about the IPA. Tellingly, and leaving his discontent in no doubt, Lacan wrote,

> the EFP (École Freudians de Paris) has nourished . . . demonstrating through acts that it is not of their doing that my Ecole would be an Institution, the effect of a consolidated group, at the expense of the discursive effect expected from an experiment, when it is Freudian. One knows what price was paid for Freud's having permitted the psychoanalytic group to win out over discourse, becoming a Church.
>
> (Lacan, 1980/1990)

Both Freud and Lacan made groups and the communal field elemental to the transmission of psychoanalysis in the full knowledge that the human race is an admixture of inhuman ferocity, discontent, and selfishness as well as endowed with qualities and potentialities such as love and sublimation that temper, humanise, and communalise. In a time when political and social speech has become increasingly hate-filled and unneighbourly, what can the psychoanalytic discourse offer? It provides a thoughtful model with which to interrogate the impossibility of any group to successfully promote the group's aims and satisfy the individual. Such a model is important, as communality is necessary to human welfare and psychical well-being and isn't going anywhere. To build in impossibility is to commit to the possible and the new in the future. While psychoanalysis has not yet provided a complete model of a successful group and is unlikely to do so, it can model the work and commitment necessary to maintain an openness to the real at the heart of all human relations. The psychoanalytic discourse is a social bond that demands something be created out of nothing.

Note

1 Notably, Carl Jung, who was Freud's own designated heir, famously split with him in 1911 and went on to establish his own group based at the Burgolzli Institute in Switzerland. Another of Freud's contemporaries, Otto Rank, developed his own theory of trauma and diverged from Freud with his experimental methods. Wilhelm Reich

was thrown out of the psychoanalytic movement in 1934 for his extreme political views. The controversial discussions about female sexuality in the 1930s were indicative of another split and resulted in Ernest Jones, Helena Deutsch, and others going their separate ways from Freud. In Lacan's case, numerous acolytes and key members of his group left his group and set up their own groups, beginning with Sasha Nacht in 1953. Piera Aulagnier, Francois Perrier, and Jean-Paul Valebrega together formed their own "fourth" group in 1969 (see Jones 1961; Roudinesco 1997; Gay 1998).

Works Cited

Cottet, S. (2012). *Freud and the Desire of the Psychoanalyst*. London: Karnac Books.

Foucault, M. (1990). *The History of Sexuality: The Will to Knowledge*, Vol. 1. London: Penguin Books.

Freud, S. (1910/2001). *The Future Prospects for Psychoanalytic Therapy*. The Standard Edition of the Complete Psychological Works of Sigmund Freud, Vol. 11, pp. 141–151. London: Vintage.

Freud, S. (1915/2001). *The Unconscious*. The Standard Edition of the Complete Psychological Works of Sigmund Freud, Vol. 14, pp. 159–215. London: Vintage.

Freud, S. (1917/2001). *Mourning and Melancholia*. The Standard Edition of the Complete Psychological Works of Sigmund Freud, Vol. 14, pp. 243–260. London: Vintage.

Freud, S. (1921/2001). *Group Psychology and the Analysis of the Ego*. The Standard Edition of the Complete Psychological Works of Sigmund Freud, Vol. 18, pp. 65–143. London: Vintage.

Freud, S. (1929/2001). *Civilization and Its Discontents*. The Standard Edition of the Complete Psychological Works of Sigmund Freud, Vol. 21, pp. 59–145. London: Vintage.

Gabriel, T. (2021, January 7). "Trump's Fights Are Their Fights: They Have his Back Unapologetically." *The New York Times*. See www.nytimes.com/2020/08/25/us/politics/trump-reelection-supporters.html.

Gay, P. (1998). *Freud: A Life for Our Time*. London and New York: W.W. Norton & Co.

Hofstein, F. (2010). "The Institution of Lacan." *Group: A Journal of the Eastern Group Psychotherapy Society*. Special Issue on Jacques Lacan and Group Psychotherapy 34(2).

Jones, E. (1961). *The Life and Work of Sigmund Freud*. Edited & Unbridged. London: Penguin Books.

Lacan, J. (1949/2006). "The Mirror Stage as Formative of the I Function as Revealed Psychoanalytic Experience." In *Ècrits: The First Complete Edition in English*. Trans. B. Fink, pp. 75–81. London: W.W. Norton & Co.

Lacan, J. (1956/2006). "The Situation of Psychoanalysis and the Training of Psychoanalysts in 1956." In *Ècrits: The First Complete Edition in English*. Trans. B. Fink, pp. 384–411. London: W.W. Norton & Co.

Lacan, J. (1964/2004). *The Seminar of Jacques Lacan Book, Book XI, The Four Fundamental Concepts of Psycho-Analysis*. London: Karnac.

Lacan, J. (1964/2006). "The Position of the Unconscious." In *Ècrits: The First Complete Edition in English*. Trans. B. Fink, pp. 703–721. London: W.W. Norton & Co.

Lacan, J. (1964-65). *Crucial Problems in Psychoanalysis*. Trans. C. Gallagher. See http://www.lacaninireland.com/web/wp-content/uploads/2010/06/12-Crucial-problems-for-psychoanalysis.pdf.

Lacan, J. (1967). *Proposal of 9 October 1967 on the Psychoanalyst of the School*. Trans. C. Gallagher. See www.lacaninireland.com/web/wp-content/uploads/2010/06/Proposal-of-the-analyst-of-the-school-1967.pdf.

Lacan, J. (1967–68/2008). "My Teaching, Its Nature and Its Ends." In *My Teaching*, pp. 57–89. London: Verso

Lacan, J. (1980). *The Seminar of Jacques Lacan Book XXVII: Dissolution*. Unpublished.

Lacan, J. (1980/1990). "Letter of Dissolution." In *Television: A Challenge to the Psychoanalytic Establishment*. London: W.W. Norton & Co.

LaFrance, A. (2020, June). "The Prophecies of Q: American Conspiracy Theories are Entering a Dangerous New Phase." In *The Atlantic*, Issue. See www.theatlantic.com/magazine/archive/2020/06/qanon-nothing-can-stop-what-is-coming/610567/.

Lewis, A. (2000). "From the Work of Transference to the Transference to the Work." *Analysis* 9.

Lewis, T. (2021, January 11). "The 'Shared Psychosis' of Donald Trump and his Loyalists." In *Scientific American*. See www.scientificamerican.com/article/the-shared-psychosis-of-donald-trump-and-his-loyalists/.

Philips, A. (2014). *Becoming Freud: The Making of a Psychoanalyst*. London and New Haven: Yale University Press.

Roudinesco, E. (1997). *Jacques Lacan*. Cambridge, UK: Polity Press.

Safouan, M. (2000). *Jacques Lacan and the Question of Psychoanalytic Training*. Trans, J. Rose. Basingstoke and London: MacMillan.

Safouan, M. (2003, November). "On the Formation of the Psychoanalyst." Talk delivered in Strasbourg.

Chapter 10

A Spectral Materialism to Safeguard Modernity

Tractatus Economico-Psychanalytico-Philosophicus

Alireza Taheri

1 A strict measure of exclusion inaugurates the attempt to forge modernity.

1.1 Kant (1929) warns against reason's conceit to confront metaphysical questions such as those concerning:

- The limits (or lack thereof) of time and space.
- The divisibility or indivisibility of matter.
- Free will and determinism.
- The existence of God.

1.11 For Kant, the attempt to delve into these noumenal matters leads to the impasse of the *antinomies of reason*.

1.12 Thought would henceforth have to limit itself to the sober domain of science defined as the study of phenomena – how things *appear* rather than how they are *in-themselves* (noumena).

1.2 This measure of exclusion, intended to protect and guarantee the advent of the modern, paradoxically leads to the failure of modernity's realization.

1.21 The inaugural exclusion by which modernity attempts to establish itself leads to a *return of the repressed* compromising modernity's fulfilment.

1.22 Such resurgences of the pre-modern within our contemporary late modernity are attested to by the rise of New Age spirituality, the proliferation of new religiosities, the obscurantism of modern American psychiatry and the mystical faith in the "invisible hand of the market".

2 By contrast to the Kantian banishment of the noumenal, Hegel, Marx and Freud dare to grant attention to tabooed objects relegated to premodern concern by Kant.

2.1 Hegel revives interest in the noumenal, claiming that the aim of his *Science of Logic* is nothing less than "the exposition of God as he is in

DOI: 10.4324/9781003212072-11

his eternal essence before the creation of nature and a finite mind" (Hegel, 1969, 50).

2.2 Marx centres his critique of classical political economy on an analysis of the "metaphysical subtleties and theological niceties" (Marx, 2000, 50) of commodities.

2.3 Freud returns to the dream – formerly the passion of fortune tellers and soothsayers – as the "royal road to the unconscious" (Freud, 1900).

2.4 It is only by returning to these forsaken objects as well as other "spectral" entities (Derrida, 2006) that modernity can forge for itself an unshakable materialism immune to the resurgences of pre-modern superstition.

3 The paradox of modernity states that we must return to these objects of pre-modern occupation in order to become modern.

3.1 The common understanding cannot fathom this paradox, and this failure of thought results in the resurgence of the pre-modern within modernity.

3.2 Since the safeguarding of the modern requires returning the gaze on objects of the pre-modern, science alone is not sufficient on our path to completing the project of modernity.

3.21 The "spectral fields" (psychoanalysis, Marxism and Hegelian speculative philosophy) are the required next steps to safeguard the modern.[1]

3.321 Without this next step beyond the limits of science, we are the mercy of scientism, biologism, capitalism and other vagaries.

3.322 Until this next step is taken, our modernity will continue to be marked by *the battle of pure prestige*[2] between a prevailing scientific attitude and an opposed spiritualist or "intuitive" attitude.

3.3221 Neither the scientific nor the spiritualist attitude can provide a *materialist* account of the spectral.

3.32211 When the spectral is (not) accounted for by the scientific attitude, we are relegated to the scientism (e.g. "modern" American psychiatry).

3.32212 When the spectral is (not) accounted for by the spiritual attitude, we regress to pre-modern superstition as in the prevailing New Age movement.

3.3222 The late modern conceptual battle of pure prestige involves a conflict between two attitudes that cannot fathom that they share in common the obfuscation of the paradoxical category of the material-spectral.

3.323 The spectral fields, by contrast, absolve the false dichotomy of mind and matter, the spiritual and the material.

3.3231 The spectral fields refrain from unnecessarily opting for one side of this false dualism in favour of the other.

3.32311 Brute simple-minded materialism chooses the material while obscurantist superstition engages in empty spirituality.

3.323111 Both of these insufficient choices miss the idea that the so-called spiritual is the (non)-point of torsion within the material.

3.3231111 The notion of the spectral names this symptomatic (non)-point.

4 The move to the spectral fields requires a transition from causal thinking to symptom-thinking.[3]

4.1 The spectral is the symptomatic and the symptomatic is the spectral.
4.2 The symptom is not an irrational oddity, marring an otherwise perfect rationality.
4.3 The symptom is hyper-rational.

4.31 Quipping Hegel, we may say, *what is hyper-rational is the symptom and, conversely, that which is a symptom is hyper-rational.*
4.32 The symptomatic torsion on the Mobius strip is not the insignia of unreason but, rather, the sign of reason's hyper-presence.[4]

4.4 To grapple with infinite spirit, the realm of human striving and consciousness, requires symptom-thinking.[5]

4.41 Nietzsche's gargantuan *revaluation of all values* rested on the achievement of symptom-thinking in the realm of morality.

4.411 "After all, today at least we immoralists have the suspicion that the decisive value of an action lies precisely in what is *unintentional* in it, while everything about it that is intentional, everything about it that can be seen, known, 'conscious,' still belongs to its surface and skin – which, like every skin, betrays something but *conceals* even more. In short, we believe that the intention is merely a sign and symptom that still requires interpretation – moreover, a sign that means too much and therefore, taken by itself alone, almost nothing" (Nietzsche, 2000, 234).

4.42 Marx achieved symptom-thinking in the realm of economics and social thought.

4.421 Lacan (2006) thus credits Marx for inventing the symptom.

4.43 Freud achieved symptom-thinking in the realm of psychology.

4.431 Freud's biologism is a retreat ("*fourvoiement*", as Laplanche (1999) calls it) from symptom-thinking.

4.44 Hegel's notion of the *absolute* heralds the Marxist and Freudian notions of the symptom.

4.441 Hegel pushed beyond Kantian formalism and abstract universality in order to grapple with the complexities of human (infinite) spirit.[6]

5 In his exploration of medieval political theology, Ernst Kantorowicz (1985) argues that the feudal kings of yesteryear were conceptualized as having two bodies:

- A material biological body.
- A body transformed by the royal title and sovereign position conferred to the subject.

5.1 Following this argument, Eric Santner (2011) holds that the modern subject, by virtue of the sovereignty gained in modernity, is also divided between a biological body and a body altered through symbolic investiture.

5.11 For both the sovereign king and the modern subject, a second body emerges as a sublime or abject surplus over the material body of biology.

5.12 What matters for Hegel is the advent of infinite spirit beyond the finitude of animal becoming.

5.121 For him, it is the "sickness of the animal" that "gives birth to spirit".

5.1211 Following Hegelian diction, we could thus say that the libidinal body is the index of the sickness of the material body.

5.1212 The libidinal body is the abode of infinite spirit.

5.13 Analogously, Marx addresses the second body of merchandise.

5.131 Marx is interested in the manner through which an ordinary thing becomes a transcendent commodity.

5.132 The "theological niceties" of the commodity mark the signature of infinite spirit upon inanimate matter.

5.14 Psychoanalysis addresses the second body of the modern subject.

5.141 It conceives the body as a *libidinal* body.

6 Our pseudo-modernity fails materialism through denials of the spectral that lead to its degradation in various forms.

6.1 The psychiatric understanding the symptom in a medical sense represents a degradation of the spectral.

6.11 Modern American psychiatry ignores the spectral libidinal body in favour of the biological body; it reduces the former to the latter.

6.12 Psychiatry also reifies the symbolic Other (the spectral entity *par excellence*) to the realm of biology.

6.2 There is a degradation of the spectrality of the erotic.

6.21 The contemporary criminalization of the erotic is a massive resurgence of puritanism by which the spectral dimension of the erotic is obliterated.

6.22 The erotic is spectral and the spectral is erotic.

6.221 When the dimension of spectrality is degraded, we have desexualization.

6.2211 Desexualization involves the reduction of the spectral libidinal body to the biological body.

6.2212 Insults and profanations offer a delicious spice to the exquisite delights of the forbidden fruit. However, when these break a certain threshold, sexual tension is flattened. A joke testifies to this. A young woman tells her partner that she finds it kinky to be insulted during sex. In the midst of their next sexual encounter, he thus exclaims: "I shit on your father's grave". The lack of subtlety missed the mark of the sexual-spectral leading to either anger and tears or chuckles, two insignia of desexualization.[7]

6.222 Humour is also spectral.

6.2221 Žižek's jokes are thus to be taken with utmost earnestness as forays into and flirtations with the spectral.

6.3 Capitalism is the economic degradation of the spectral.

6.31 Commodity fetishism is essential and inevitable in capitalist political-economic life.

6.311 Bourgeois thought and classical political economy misconstrue this fetishism.
6.312 Marx recognizes that the thing acquires a second body that transforms it into a commodity.
6.313 The second body gives rise to fetishism.
6.314 When a thing of use becomes a commodity, it is changed into something transcendent (Marx, 2000, 50).

6.3141 Commodities abound in "metaphysical subtleties and theological niceties" (ibid.: 50).
6.3142 Commodities are "sensuous things which are at the same time supra-sensible or social" (Marx quoted in Harvey, 2018, 41).

6.31421 The two bodies are therefore:

- The sensuous body of the thing.
- The supra-sensible and social "body".

6.32 Commodity fetishism involves the inevitable misperception by which labour as social form is falsely reduced to the objective trait of products.

6.321 Marx speaks of "the mist through which the social character of labour appears to us to be an objective character of the products themselves" (Marx, 2000, 56).
6.322 Marx: "the commodity reflects the social characteristics of men's own labour as objective characteristics of the products of labour themselves, as the socio-natural properties of these things" (Marx quoted in Harvey, 2018, 41).

6.323 This leads to the following obfuscation: "There is a definite social relation between men, that assumes, in their eyes, the fantastic form of a relation between things" (Marx, 2000, 52).

6.324 The social association between people is the real source of the spectral gleam of the commodity.

6.3241 Labour and the relations between labourers is the ephemeral spectral entity that gives the commodity its super-sensuous metaphysical aspect.

6.3242 Fetishism, Harvey (2018) argues, is inevitable because, due to the complications of the world market, you cannot know everything about the labourers involved that constitute the social association between people.

6.33 Value is the spectral entity that arises as the congealed symptom of labour-time.

6.331 Money is the imaginary representation of the spectral (value).

6.3311 Money is a reification and hypostatization of the spectrality of value.

7 Hegel is the philosophical-theological guardian of the spectral.

7.1 For Hegel, God is the spectral entity *par excellence.*

7.2 For Hegel, the Kantian antinomies were testament not to the failure of reason but, rather, to its successful articulation of the contradictions inherent to being.

7.21 Hegel thus grasps the spectral through logic and speculative reason.

7.22 For Hegel, the spectral-spiritual is the contradictory and the contradictory is the spectral-spiritual.

7.221 The principal lesson from Hegel: being is spectral insofar as it is contradictory.

7.222 Dialectics is the Hegelian spectral field insofar as it begins with the premise that being is contradictory.

8 Marx is the economic guardian of the spectral.

8.1 Marx's style of writing in the chapter on commodity fetishism is literary rather than technical (Harvey, 2018, 40).

8.11 There are references to "magic, mysteries and necromancies" (ibid.: 40).

8.111 We are dealing with the spectral dimension.

8.1111 This may be the reason Althusser (1996) opted for a *symptomatic* reading of *Capital.*

8.2 For Marx, value is a quintessentially spectral entity.

8.21 Marx compares value to gravity: "the labour-time socially necessary to produce [commodities] asserts itself as a regulative law of nature. In the same way, the law of gravity asserts itself when a person's house collapses on top of him" (Marx quoted in Harvey, 2018, 44–45).

8.211 As Harvey puts it, gravity and value are both "relations and not things, and both have to be conceptualized as immaterial but objective" (ibid.: 2018).

8.2111 We here encounter a great definition of the spectral as the *immaterial* and *objective*.

8.2111 This is perfectly in line with the lesson learnt from Hegel, namely that the spectral is the contradictory; the contradiction here lies in the opposition between the objective and the immaterial.

8.22 Commodity fetishism involves the obliteration of the spectrality of value.

8.221 Commodity fetishism makes concrete (rather than spectral) the objectivity of value; this is the inherent hypostatization and reification of fetishism.

8.2211 Marx founds a field that avoids the fetishistic hypostatization of the spectrality of value.

8.22111 This is a spectral field that is neither scientism nor pre-modern superstition.

9 Freud and Lacan are the psychoanalytic guardians of the spectral.

9.1 The Freudian-Lacanian unconscious is spectral.

9.11 The idea of "depth-psychology" is a hypostatization of the spectral.

9.2 The clinical notion of transference names the spectral entity that haunts the analytic relation.

9.21 To reduce the transference to repetition involves a hypostatization of the spectral.

9.211 The spectrality of transference is the conduit for change.

9.22 Transference is erotic because it is spectral.

9.23 To properly handle the clinical situation requires acknowledging the spectral entity that is the transference.

9.231 The denial of this spectral presence will disparage the clinical situation to suggestion and acting out.

9.2311 Lacan's idea according to which "transference without interpretation is acting-out" (Lacan, 2004) implies that the task of interpretation is to maintain the spectral dimension of transference.

9.23111 This is achieved by maintaining interpretation on the symbolic axis linking the subject to the unconscious.

9.23112 When interpretation takes place on the imaginary axis linking the egos of the analyst and analysand, the spectral dimension of transference is reified and hypostatized.

9.231121 Acting *out* and *suggestion* are the names of the reification and hypostatization through which spectral-erotic transference is flattened.

9.2311211 Through the flattening and neutralization of the spectral, transference is either entirely desexualized or it becomes overtly erotomanic.

9.3 Paternal authority and power are spectral.

9.31 Following our Hegelian idea, we recall that the spectral is contradictory.

9.311 Paternal authority, insofar as it is spectral, is also contradictory.

9.3111 The contradiction of the spectrality of paternal power: if paternal authority is hypostatized as force, it immediately loses its power.

9.31111 Another formulation of the contradiction of spectral paternal power: paternal authority is sustained paradoxically only when it refrains from exhibiting itself and remains hidden.

9.31112 "The real in the background that serves as the ultimate guarantee and support of the public power is thus a spectral entity – not only does it not need to exist in reality, if it did appear and directly intervene in reality, then it would risk losing its power, since, as Lacan made clear, omnipotence (toute-puissance) necessarily reverts into 'all-in-potency' (tout en puissance): a father who is perceived as 'omnipotent' can only sustain this position if his power remains forever a 'potential,' a threat which is never actualized" (Žižek, 2015, 54).

9.3112 Another contradiction of paternal authority is that it represents the paradoxical dialectical unity of force and love.

9.31121 For Hegel, the punishment of children lifts "the universal into their consciousness and will" (Hegel, 2008, 173). In other words, the law requires force.

9.311211 However, this force of law must be held in dialectical unity with love.

9.311212 Punishment accompanied by love gives the child the chance to achieve true concern for the other.

9.3112121 Achieving this requires the proverbial paternal cane, but its aim is precisely to overcome the cane.

9.31121211 The paternal cane provides its own sublation; if it hits the child once, it is with the aim of never having to do so again.

9.311212111 As self-sublating, the cane is a speculative object, namely a thing of love.

9.3112121111 As speculative object, the paternal cane is, to quip Hegel, "not only as Substance, but equally as Subject" (Hegel, 1977, 10).

9.3113 Another contradiction of the paternal law (and the law in general) is that its expression must be held in dialectical unity with its dissolution and disappearance.

9.31131 The *voice* of the law must disappear so that its message is received (Lebrun, 1972, 298–299).

9.311311 Lebrun refers to Hegel's notion of *expression*, referring to a presence that is inseparable from dissolution (ibid.: 298).

9.3113111 The leap of faith testifying to acceptance of the paternal law (symbolic castration) will not take place if the voice carrying it persists beyond its message.

9.3114 Another contradiction of the law is that, for Hegel, a criminal act is its own punishment.

9.31141 To separate the two moments of crime and punishment is to suffer of the ideology of time that unnecessarily separates temporally the two moments of a given dialectical unity.[8]

9.311411 Thus, the wisest operation of the law is to let the crime be its own punishment.

9.3114111 Once this intractable dialectical unity is achieved, penance and expiation will be reached.

9.4 The dream is the "royal road" to the spectral.

9.41 As such, the dream must be dealt with extreme care to avoid hypostatization and reification.

9.411 The contemporary resistance to psychoanalysis has led to two forms of the hypostatization of the dream.

9.4111 The first involves the scientistic relegation of the dream to meaningless non-sense.

9.4112 The second involves the obscurantist elevation of the dream to oracle or divination (New Ageism and Jungianism).

9.5 The Freudian-Lacanian notion of the Other also points to a spectral entity that is at once immaterial and objective.

9.51 The so-called big Other is an "objective order" emerging "out of the interaction of individuals" and "experienced by the individuals involved as a substantial agency which determines their lives" (Žižek, 2012, 972).

9.52 The Other is a constitutive spectral presence in the community of human speakers and is, as such, ineradicable.

9.521 Hegel presciently makes the point regarding the ineradicability of the Other in the following notable passage: "The educational experiments, advocated by Rousseau in Émile, of withdrawing people from the common life of every day and bringing them up in the country, have turned out to be futile, since no success can attend an attempt to estrange people from the laws of the world. Even if the young have to be educated in solitude, one should still not imagine that the fragrance of the spiritual world will not ultimately permeate this solitude or that the power of the world spirit is too feeble to gain mastery of those outlying regions. It is by becoming a citizen of a good state that the individual first comes into his right" (Hegel, 2008, 160–161).

9.5111 The remarkable notion of "the fragrance of the spiritual world" beautifully evokes the idea of an immaterial existence that is nonetheless objective.

9.53 The spectral Other is hypostatized in psychosis but is not eradicated.

9.531 The delusions of paranoia involve nothing other than the hypostatization of the spectral Other into a given person or group of people.

9.532 The auditory and visual hallucinations of psychosis involve the hypostatization of the spectral Other into signifiers returning in the real to haunt the subject.

9.533 In psychotic depression or melancholia, the spectral Other is reified as the shadow of the object (Freud, 1917) that falls on the subject's ego.

9.534 When the Other is hypostatized, it becomes for the subject a privileged locus of projections leading to a specular imaginary relation with the Other.

9.535 In religion, the Other is reified into God.

9.5351 As Lacan has noted, "the God hypothesis" (Lacan, 1998, 45) will always persist.

9.536 Subjective responsibility involves resisting the urge to hypostatize the Other and thereby avoiding the specular relation that would follow.

9.5361 This requires the speculative feat of recognizing that the spectral Other is the result of the subject's self-reflection.

9.53611 The Hegelian *beautiful soul*[9] cannot grasp the paradox that the Other is the result of his/her own self-reflection.

9.53612 That the Other is the result of the subject's self-reflection means that the Other is nothing other than how it is *perceived*, and to this we must add, moreover, that the Other is perceived in accordance to the subject's own manner of perceiving.

9.536121 This bizarre tautology means that the Other is the reflection of the subject's own gaze.

9.536122 The subject will relate in his/her own way to this Other or, more accurately, the subject will *constitute* this Other in accordance to his/her own subject position.

9.5361221 Thus, "Evil resides in the gaze itself which perceives the object as Evil" (Hegel quoted in Žižek, 1998).

9.5361222 An envious gaze will render the Other envious and so on.

9.5361223 In acting out and *passage à l'acte* the spectral Other is reified and concretized as an other person.

9.53612231 Acting out involves a spectacle staged for the imagined gaze of the other person.

9.53612232 *Passage à l'acte* occurs when the other person's gaze emerges on the scene as a real spectator.

9.53613 The free and responsible subject must take cognizance of the fact that the Other is a product of his/her self-reflection, i.e. that subject and Other stand in identity-in-difference.

9.536131 This is why the psychoanalytic cure involves nothing more than a slight shift of perspective, a turn as subtle as the near-indiscernible torsion on the Mobius strip.

9.5361311 The cure marks the moment of the paradoxical dialectical unity of the infinitesimal shift and the infinite transformation.

9.53614 The free and responsible subject must take cognizance of the fact that the Other is a product of his/her self-reflection, i.e. that subject and Other stand in identity-in-difference.

9.536141 As in game theory and structural anthropology, psychoanalysis does not care for the "character", "personality" or "depth" of the individual.

9.5361411 Psychoanalysis is interested only in the position the subject takes up in relation to the spectral Other and, moreover, how that position constitutes the Other for the subject.

9.53614111 Psychoanalysis is also interested in the jouissance that that position renders for the subject.

9.53614112 With a change effected through interpretation, psychoanalysis hopes to bring a change in:

- The subject's position vis-à-vis the Other.
- The Other as it is constituted by the subject's position.
- The *jouissance* rendered by the relation of the subject to the Other.

10 The true meaning of materialism is: to view "metaphysical" things (the Other, language, God, miracles, ghosts, value, medical symptoms) in neither a spiritual nor a scientistically reductive manner.

10.1 Ignoring the spectral altogether is tantamount to scientism.

10.2 Resorting to spiritual explanations involves the pre-modern hypostasis of otherworldly realms.

10.3 The tightrope upon which we walk is situated precisely between arrogant scientism and ignorant obscurantism.

10.31 We are accompanied by topology on this tightrope; it tells us that the spectre is nothing other than the torsion on the surface creating the illusion of height and the fear that we may *fall*.

10.4 As harbingers of the modernity to come, we face the challenge of the following speculative proposition: *the spectral is the material and, conversely, the material is the spectral.*

10.5 The spectral resists the reifications and hypostatizations of pseudo-modernity.

11 Hegel, Marx, Freud and Lacan provide the spectral antidote to reification/hypostatization in the form of a *symptomatic* point.

11.1 From the perspective they have opened, we may conclude that the symptom is the spectral-materialist antidote to reification and hypostatization.

11.2 Hegel christens the symptomatic point as *absolute.*

11.21 The symptomatic point is a locus of protest against reification.

11.3 For Freud and Lacan, the symptomatic point takes the form of lapses in speech, dreams and quotidian errors as so many testaments to the unconscious.

11.31 The symptomatic point is a locus of protest against the Other.

11.4 For Marx, the labour power of the proletariat is the symptomatic point of the capitalist mode of production.

11.41 Social movements (led by the proletariat) provide the locus of protest against the dominance of politics and economics.

12 When Hegel claims that "everything turns on grasping and expressing the True, not only as Substance, but equally as Subject" (Hegel, 1977, 10), he expresses the limitation of abstract formalism.

12.1 This recalcitrant resistance to abstract universality is the signature of the human, the entity that most stubbornly defies its definition.

12.11 Neuroscience and genetics also argue that the human being is genetically programmed to defy its genetic programming (cf. Ansermet and Magistretti, 2004).

12.2 The symptom – the marker of discomfort par excellence – testifies to the human madness that contests most explicitly all formalism (Taheri, 2021, 150).

12.21 The symptom provides the *notion of human* and is, as such, the antidote to abstract universality.

13 The spectral fields of Hegelian speculative philosophy, Marxism and psychoanalysis carry an important ethical mandate, namely to *identify with the symptom.*

13.1 Such an achievement is the height of the speculative paradox by which the human and the inhuman stand in identity-in-difference.

13.11 At the individual level, this consists of the abolition of the ego.

13.111 Lacan christens this as *subjective destitution.*

13.12 At the social level, this consists of revolution through which social movements contest the hegemony of the political and the economic order.

13.121 Marx christens this as the dictatorship of the proletariat.

Notes

1 Althusser (2006) spoke of psychoanalysis and Marxism as "conflictual sciences". Despite its partial validity, such a designation already involves an unnecessary imaginarization of the spectral. More accurately, psychoanalysis and Marxism (as well as Hegel's speculative philosophy) are fields concerned with the spectral real. The conceptualization of a conflict with an Other always involves a degradation of the real to the imaginary where internal division is (mis)-perceived as external strife.

2 The notion of a *battle of pure prestige* comes from Kojève's (1980) return to Hegel's (1977) master–slave dialectic. It denotes a battle between two conscious human beings for domination regardless of the risk it may pose to their own life. I use the term to designate any dual conflict where the partisans care more for triumph than the truth and where they are blind to the fact that they speak from the same subject position as the rival whom they critique.

3 The exact nature of this transition is beyond the scope of the present chapter and will constitute a central concern of my next book.

4 The propositions from 4.1 to 4.32 are ideas from my *Hegelian-Lacanians Variations on Late Modernity: Spectre of Madness* (*Conclusion: From via dolorosa to gaya scienza*).

5 Hegel makes use of the terms finite and infinite spirit to refer, respectively, to nature at large and the realm of the specifically human. It is arguable that he also holds that the inanimate and plant and animal realms already hold the kernel of infinite spirit within them. This follows from the fact that absolute knowing, for Hegel, is there from the start rather than representing an endpoint. Thus, regarding the "True", Hegel says that it is "the process of its own becoming, the circle that presupposes its end as its goal, having its end also as its beginning" (Hegel, 1977, 10).

6 Hegel asserts, against Kant, that formalism "imagines that it has comprehended and expressed the nature and life of a form when it has endowed it with some determination of the schema as a predicate" (Hegel, 1977, 29). For Hegel, the attempt to impose generalizations such as "laws of nature" on particulars fails to appreciate that that "everything turns on grasping and expressing the True, not only as Substance, but equally as Subject" (ibid.: 10).

7 I make use of this joke in (Taheri, 2021) as well (cf. *Variation 13: Sexual Difference: Man and Woman*).

8 The propositions from 9.31111 to 9.3114 are ideas from my *Hegelian-Lacanians Variations on Late Modernity: Madness* (*Variation 19: The Force and Frailty of the Law*).

9 Hegel uses this term to designate the subject who cannot appreciate his/her complicity in the situation that he/she bemoans.

Works Cited

Althusser, L. (1996) *Lire Le Capital*. Quadrige. PUF.

Althusser, L. (2006) *For Marx*. Translated by Brewster, B. Verso.

Ansermet, F. and Magistretti, P. (2004) *À chacun son cerveau: plasticité neuronale et inconscient*. Odile Jacob.

Derrida, J. (2006) *Specters of Marx. The State of the Debt, the Work of Mourning and the New International*. Routledge.

Freud, S. (1900) *The Interpretation of Dreams. The Standard Edition of the Complete Psychological Works of Sigmund Freud*. Translated by Strachey, J. Vintage, the Hogarth Press. S.E. 4.

Freud, S. (1917) *Mourning and Melancholia. The Standard Edition of the Complete Psychological Works of Sigmund Freud*. Translated by Strachey, J. Vintage, the Hogarth Press. S.E. 14.

Harvey, D. (2018) *A Companion to Marx's Capital. The Complete Edition*. Verso.

Hegel, G.W.F. (1969) *Science of Logic*. Translated by Miller, A.V. Foreword by Findlay, J.N. Humanity Books, an imprint of Prometheus Books.

Hegel, G.W.F. (1977) *Phenomenology of Spirit*. Translated by Miller, A.V. With analysis of the text and foreword by Findlay, J.N. Oxford University Press.

Hegel, G.W.F. (2008) *Outlines of the Philosophy of Right*. Oxford University Press.

Kant, I. (1929) *Critique of Pure Reason*. Translated by Smith, N.K. Macmillan (reissue St. Martin's Press, 1965).

Kantorowicz, E. (1985) *The King's Two Bodies. A Study in Medieval Political Theology*. Princeton University Press.

Kojève, A. (1980) *Introduction à la lecture de Hegel*. Gallimard.

Lacan, J. (1998) *The Seminar of Jacques Lacan. Book XX. Encore* (1972–1973). Translated with notes by Fink, B. W.W Norton & Company. New York and London.

Lacan, J. (2004) *Le séminaire. Livre X. L'angoisse*. Le Seuil.

Lacan, J. (2006) *Écrits*. Translated by Fink, B. In collaboration with Fink, H. and Grigg, R.W. W.W. Norton and Company.

Laplanche, J. (1999) *La sexualité humaine, biologisme et biologie*. Institut Synthélabo. Le Plessis-Robinson.

Lebrun, G. (1972) *La Patience du concept: Essai sur le discours hégélien*. Gallimard.

Marx, K. (2000) *Das Kapital. A Critique of Political Economy*. Edited by Engels, F. and condensed by Levitsky, S. A Gateway Edition. Regnery Gateway.

Nietzsche, F. (2000) *Beyond Good and Evil*. Translated and edited by Kaufmann, W. Basic Writings of Nietzsche. The Modern Library.

Santner, E. (2011) *The Royal Remains: The People's Two Bodies and the Endgames of Sovereignty*. University of Chicago Press.

Taheri, A. (2021) *Hegelian-Lacanians Variations on Late Modernity: Spectre of Madness*. Routledge.

Žižek, S. (1998) "For a Leftist Appropriation of the European Legacy" in *Journal of Political Ideologies*. February, 1998.

Žižek, S. (2012) *Less Than Nothing: Hegel and the Shadow of Dialectical Materialism*. Verso Books.

Žižek, S. (2015) *Absolute Recoil: Towards a New Foundation of Dialectical Materialism*. Verso Books.

Chapter 11

Invisible Fist of the Market

Fight Club and the Therapeutic Lures of Violence

Daniel Adleman

Chuck Palahniuk's *Fight Club* is often mischaracterized as an uncritical celebration of misogynistic proto-incel terrorism. This critique is somewhat understandable given the alt-right's notorious uptake of the term "snowflake," an epithet that derives from Tyler Durden's oratory in the novel and David Fincher's popular film adaptation. Against the grain of popular misconceptions, I argue the novel is best understood as a nuanced, ambivalent interrogation of conventional understandings of violence. Far from blithely celebrating the indiscriminate violence of fight clubs, Palahniuk's novel documents the flawed, therapeutic pilgrim's progress of its nameless protagonist, whom some literary critics call "Joe," to channel and remediate the systemic violence of post-Fordist neoliberal capitalism in politically emancipatory directions.

This chapter explores the psychoanalytic dimensions of Joe's increasingly entangled therapeutic and activist strategies to metabolize and wield what he explicitly characterizes as the castrating paternal violence of corporate-colonized America. His ever-unfolding odyssey to save himself and others (through his experiments with terminal disease self-help groups, fight clubs, anti-corporate activism, and ultimately terrorism) sheds light on the complex roles of different modalities of violence in late capitalist society. The author concludes by bringing some of these perspectives on violence into resonance with contemporary protest movements like Occupy Wall Street and Idle No More.

Sleepless Nights of Labour

Fight Club begins with a listless Joe seeking out medical treatment for his deep-seated insomnia. A medical practitioner advises him, "insomnia is just the symptom of something larger. Find out what's actually wrong. Listen to your body" (19). In "A Generation of Men Without History," Krister Friday cites the doctor's advice as "paradigmatic for the text's overt interest

DOI: 10.4324/9781003212072-12

in masculine affliction and its etiology." (Friday 5). "What the narrator discovers," writes Friday, "is that this 'something larger' is a crisis of masculinity in contemporary American culture – a crisis that produces conspicuous symptoms and necessitates even more conspicuous remedies" (Friday 5). I contend that this succession of "conspicuous symptoms" and ad hoc remedies unfurls in accordance with a political–psychoanalytic logic that requires meticulous unpacking.

Joe's household is a much-overlooked but conspicuous locus of his uneasiness. He lives in a hermetically sealed high-rise condominium, which he describes as "a sort of *filing cabinet* for widows and young professionals" (41), about which he muses:

> The marketing brochure promised a foot of concrete floor, ceiling, and wall between me and any adjacent stereo or turned-up television. A foot of concrete and air conditioning, you couldn't open the windows so even with maple flooring and dimmer switches, all seventeen hundred airtight feet would smell like the last meal you cooked or your last trip to the bathroom.
>
> (41)

As a diffident, rule-obeying consumer, Joe has installed himself in an immunized dwelling that is putatively insulated against unwelcome intrusions from the outside, including from his neighbours (many of whom dwell in their own vacuum-packed filing cabinets). And yet, his solipsistic dwelling is homogenously consubstantial with his workplace; it is a "filing cabinet" for "young professionals." Though individual others are unwelcome, the Lacanian Big Other has contoured and regulated every iota of his abode.

Joe characterizes himself as a "slave to [his] nesting instinct" (43), and he has filled his filing cabinet with corporate merchandise. In this regard, his effeminization is evidently in accordance with the consumer zeitgeist: "The people [he] know[s] who used to sit in the bathroom with pornography, now they sit in the bathroom with their IKEA furniture catalogue" (43). His account of the contemporary upending of masculine gender roles and sexuality figures his lifestyle as indentured to an effete neoliberal order. That the Ikea catalogue has supplanted the role that pornography once played in a prescriptive masculine psychic ecology bespeaks the fact that his relationship with consumerism is one of overwhelming fetishistic disavowal: his literally fetishistic relationship with consumerism staves off instincts and ideas that undermine the integrity of the American dream machine.

Not only does this new libidinal economy (if we take "economy" in a very literal sense of the term) effectively emasculate Joe, the would-be rugged male, it constitutes the very crucible of his shallow subjectivity by inserting him into an interminable circuit of product choices. Bülent

Diken and Carsten Laustsen refer to the neoliberal network of prefab consumer opportunities as a kaleidoscopic "pseudo-freedom" (Diken and Laustsen 4) of choice between equally generic consumer goods patched together into a supposedly primrose path to the Good Life.[1] In the world of *Fight Club*, the constrictive circuit of these goods operates within a broader milieu putatively conforming to Bill Gates' ideal of "friction-free capitalism." Paradoxically, this rigid network creates the illusion of unprecedented freedom, mobility, and individuality while reducing the coordinates of that freedom to the passive consumption of generic corporate-branded commodities.

The flipside of Joe's passive consumption under illusory conditions of free choice is a heightened susceptibility to, and even an uncanny ventriloquism by, the algorithmic logic of the culture industry. Picking up and elaborating on threads in the work of Adorno and Horkheimer, David Simmons and Nicola Allen describe the contemporary culture industry as "a system predicated on a fascist desire to move towards the complete homogenization of the individual" (Simmons and Allen 116). This fascistic dynamic reduces Joe to a liquidated subject, a "castrated" instrument of capital that has been trained to pursue the Good Life through proper regimens of consumption. In spite of the banality of his "nesting instinct," Joe's emasculation at the hands of the culture industry is not without psychotic side-effects. This cultural castration leads to the monstrous transfiguration of his desire, volition, and imagination in an emerging cybernetic society of control.

Lynn Ta sees Joe's form of life as a flashpoint of the contemporary American "transition from a manufacture-based economy to an information-based market, . . . transforming white middle-class working men from a vehicle of production to a womanish receptacle of consumption" (Ta 266). Expressing a measure of reflexivity about his life of ostensive effeminacy and enslavement to the marketplace, Joe reflects, "it took my whole life to buy this stuff. My Steg nesting tables. You buy furniture. . . . The drapes. The rug. Then you're trapped in your lovely nest, and the things you used to own, now they own you" (44). Slowly, insidiously, he has become imprisoned by the products of his "freedom," and it dawns on him that the consumer goods meant to complete him, while insulating him from over-proximity to the bodily lives of others, actually exercise an uncanny power over his life. Joe's assertion that "the things you used to own, now they own you" radiates out of the undead animation that haunts his "nest" and suggests his awakening to the emasculating autoimmune operations of his protective consumer bubble. In other words, his narrative arc figures as a locus of broader epistemic stirrings, including a rapidly changing libidinal marketplace at the turn of the millennium. It should come as no surprise, then, that his psychotic itinerary is, in large part, organized around (e)rectifying this disorder and reasserting his wounded manhood.

Death by Consumption

Later in the novel, looking back on his trajectory, Joe remarks,

> I hated my life. I was tired and bored with my job and my furniture, and I couldn't see any way to change things. Only end them. I felt trapped. I was too complete. I was too perfect. I wanted a way out of my tiny life. (172–173)

As an unwitting adherent of the Anna Freud school of ego psychology,[2] Joe has half-consciously set out an impossible task for himself: he has endeavoured to employ the prescriptive affordances of his late capitalist milieu in the service of achieving an unattainable state of egoic integrity. The resulting constriction of his ego-insulating experiential universe is manifold. He conducts his life in self-enclosed "filing cabinet[s]" that induce an overriding experience of solitude and autonomy, even in a large city swarming with people.[3] But, more broadly speaking, his domicile merely indexes the extent to which his pre-scripted life is cosmically insignificant and without grander purpose. Without telos or rudder, his pathologically normative lifestyle is simply that of "a cubicle-dwelling, catalog-reading, condominium-dwelling consumer" (Kavadlo 106).

In direct opposition to ego psychology, Jacques Lacan criticizes egoic fortification as a therapeutic strategy. "The ego," he writes, "is structured exactly like a symptom. At the heart of the subject, it is only a privileged symptom, the human symptom par excellence, the mental illness of man" (*Seminar I* 16). *Fight Club* seems to stage and narrativize the pitfalls of the sort of ego-buttressing strategies that consumer capitalism seduces atomized media consumers into adopting. From this standpoint, Joe's hollowed-out "filing cabinet" lifeworld is not merely mundane and innocuous; it is the fragile reification of an insidiously vicious world, whose binding logic perpetrates immense harm on his psyche.

While Joe's entire form of life has been organizing around fabricating egoic strategies that protect him from the infiltration of a violent world, his prophylactic architecture actually mediates and beams in the world in a pathological fashion. It should come as no surprise that spectres rush in to fill the void of his hollow, automated lifeworld. His sterile habitat is therefore, paradoxically, also psychotropically simulacral. As Joe descends into a somnambulistic torpor, the mimetic logic of consumer culture takes root in his psyche, rendering all "common-sensical" empirical experience "so far away, a copy of a copy of copy" (97). In "Revolutionary Bodies in Chuck Palahniuk's *Fight Club*," Olivia Burgess writes, "much like the mass-produced goods that typify his society, the narrator feels increasingly removed from an unmediated and fully experienced existence" (Burgess 270). As a desubjectified vehicle of capital, Joe is so deracinated that only a brutal rupture could afford any measure of critical distance toward the fantasy system in which he is entangled. However, as his pilgrim's progress unfolds, he discovers that not all such ruptures are emancipatory.

But there is another stratum of alienation and brutality folded into Joe's commodifying and commodified form of life. As a recall coordinator for an insurance company, his job is to callously monetize life and death according to a "liability formula":

> Wherever I'm going, I'll be there to apply the formula. I'll keep the secret intact.
>
> It's simple arithmetic.
>
> It's a story problem.
>
> If a new car built by my company leaves Chicago traveling west at 60 miles per hour, and the rear differential locks up, and the car crashes and burns with everyone trapped inside, does my company initiate a recall?
>
> You take the population of vehicles in the field (*A*) and multiply it by the probable rate of failure (*B*), then multiply the result by the average cost of an out-of-court settlement (*C*).
>
> *A* times *B* times *C* equals *X*. This is what it will cost if we don't initiate a recall.
>
> If *X* is greater than the cost of a recall, we recall the cars and no one gets hurt.
>
> If *C* is less than the cost of a recall, then we don't recall.
>
> Everywhere I go, there's the burned-up wadded-up shell of a car waiting for me. I know where all the skeletons are. Consider this my job security.
>
> (30–31)

Though Joe's empirical experience of his ego-fortifying capitalist milieu has been hitherto "peaceful" and seamless, his fantasmatic "story problem" starts to unravel. This is because it becomes increasingly difficult to fetishistically disavow the fact that he works for a voraciously "profit-driven and casually murderous corporation" (Burgess 271). "This dehumanizing and callous treatment of human life," writes Burgess,

> is indicative of a society where people are only as valuable as their capacity to consume. As an accommodating consumer, the Narrator buys stuff for his apartment, ending up in the same situation as everyone else in his or her "lovely nest."
>
> (270)

Nonetheless, he can compartmentalize his life for only so long before his own complicity in the necropolitical violence of predatory capitalism irrupts to the surface of his experience.

Narcissistic Wounds

The spiritual hollowness from which Joe suffers is the direct consequence of his world's *tout-court* colonization by the spirit of corporate consumerism. In "Acting Out Is the Best Defense in *Fight Club*," Laurie Vickroy contends that Joe's feeling of emptiness is a symptom of post-traumatic stress disorder. But, as a docile worker bee, Joe has not been sufficiently cognizant of the traumas he has absorbed as a consequence of the systemic and symbolic forms of violence folded into his subjectively peaceful milieu. The most devastating of these is his occupation as an automobile recall coordinator that is "exposed to potentially traumatic information such as . . . seeing people's legs cut off by exploding turbo chargers that the negligent company will not replace" (Vickroy 64). His vantage point affords a uniquely horrific perspective on the reification and excrementalization of human life within a necropolitical matrix that viciously reduces consumers to lifeless numbers in the actuarial data stream. This turns out to be an acutely schismatic position for him to occupy: he is simultaneously a law-abiding consumer-victim and a violent law-manipulating corporate-perpetrator of the same sinister life-monetizing corporate algorithm. He has, in a very real sense, been perpetrating harm on himself.

Joe's fragile sense of self-integrity and self-esteem, the belief that he is a "unique snowflake," is hypermediated and, therefore, completely generic. Tyler complains, "we've all been raised on television to believe that one day we'd all be millionaires and movie stars and rock stars, but we won't. And we're just learning that fact" (166). Universalizing his own contingent upbringing, he asserts that the main reason why his generation was "raised on television" is that their fathers were absent from their lives. On this point, Joe muses,

> me, I knew my dad for about six years, but I don't remember anything. My dad, he starts a new family in a new town about every six years. This isn't so much like a family as it's like he sets up a *franchise*. What you see at fight club is a generation of men raised by women.
>
> (50; my emphasis)

Acutely aware of this decline in paternal authority and mentorship, he has, on various occasions, attempted to rectify the matter by gleaning patriarchal wisdom from his absent father:

> After college, I called him long distances and said, now what? My dad didn't know. When I got a job and turned twenty-five, long distance, I said, now what? My dad didn't know, so he said, get married. I'm a thirty-year-old boy, and I'm wondering if another woman is really the answer I need.
>
> (50)

Stuck in a *disenfranchised* rut, Joe is caught up in just the kind of orphaned predicament Tyler decries: "Advertising has these people chasing cars and clothes they don't need. Generations have been working in jobs they hate, just so they can buy what they don't really need" (53). Tyler's oratory seems to anticipate the anti-capitalist rhetoric of Occupy Wall Street *avant la lettre*. But his remedy to Joe's narcissistic wound remains both slavish (in its adherence to the law of the father) and hopelessly contaminated by an almost proto-incel misogyny; and these stumbling blocks will impede its communitarian potentials.

All-Too-Human New Age Panaceas

Joe anxiously perceives his fatherless world as rudderless, effeminate, materialistic, and simulacral. The alienated agitation that undulates through his life manifests itself in his insomnia. His doctor flippantly suggests that he visit some local illness support groups in order to see people in "real pain." Taking this advice seriously, he pays them a visit in order to elucidate his own privileged circumstances. He is, however, shocked to discover that he is able to derive subterranean support from the groups, which apply a soothing balm to his emasculated, dehumanized spirit.

In "Remaining Men Together," a testicular cancer survivors' group, Joe discovers a therapeutic outlet in the company of his fellow emasculated men. Because the group underscores the fallibility and imperfection of the male body (as opposed to the generic "stock bodies" valorized by the culture industry), he is finally able to express what he experiences as human emotions. In the loving embrace of other men, he finds himself capable of shedding tears and purging the affective toxins that have welled up inside of him. "The support groups provide a temporary 'cure' for Joe, whose fleeting escapes from dominant society recharge his excitement for life," writes Burgess. "Here, among the frail and outcast, he finds an alternative to the perfection or at least the pressure to maintain the appearance of perfection" (Burgess 270). The disease therapy groups (for testicular cancer, parasites, etc.) all focus on the dying body in a fashion that allows him to return his thoughts to mortality and the life of the body. "These are unpleasant aspects of embodiment, but nevertheless reminders of the body's existence," writes Burgess. "These nightly forays into death and dying allow the Narrator to create a fantasy world where he, too, is dying, and by dying he is able to continually reembrace life" (Burgess 270-271).

Importantly, within the seemingly more immediate microcosm of "Remaining Men Together," Joe is able to exhume his wounded masculinity and his empathetic humanity; that is, until Marla Singer arrives on the scene, mirroring back his own mendacity. Like Joe, Marla is a mere "faker" (35), a "tourist" (14), who is not really dying. As a result of her abrasive overproximity to his own subterfuge, he finds himself unable to achieve therapeutic catharsis in her presence:

> In this one moment, Marla's lie reflects my lie, and all I can see are lies. In the middle of all their truth. Everyone clinging and risking to share their worst fear, that their death is coming head-on and the barrel of a gun is pressed against the back of their throats. Well, Marla is smoking and rolling her eyes, and me, I'm buried under a sobbing carpet, and all of a sudden even death and dying rank right down there with plastic flowers on video as a non-event.
>
> (23)

Her intrusion reminds Joe that his pursuit of authenticity is itself a false imitation. He is not mortally ill, at least not in the sense that his fellow group members are, "but he can copy being sick. . . . [Joe] is looking to feel 'alive' in a society where life and death have become inseparable from images compounded on images, . . . plastic flowers on video" (Burgess 271). He is far from ready to look in the mirror and acknowledge his feminine ego-double, who reflects back his own defects. Achieving catharsis away from the dominion of the effeminizing mediasphere, it turns out, is not going to be as easy as locking arms with other, more legitimate castrati. Joe's brand of symbolic castration is the product of a simulacral *Unbehagen*, a pervasive late-capitalist *dis-ease*, of which his insomnia is merely a localized symptom.

Though a misogynistic Joe is quick to scapegoat Marla (and women, in general) for his acute experience of imposture, the tectonic plates underlying "Remaining Men Together" had already been rapidly in motion well before her arrival on the scene. Indeed, Marla's appearance may very well be a psychotropic product of the seismic activity at play beneath his neatly compartmentalized psychic landscape. It is important to note that, unlike David Fincher's film adaptation of *Fight Club*, Palahniuk's novel ends with the revelation that Joe is in a mental hospital and the very strong suggestion that everything about his account, including Marla's existence, is unreliable. It is therefore surprising that many critics are so credulous to her reality, even viewing her as Joe's paramount, however tenuous, "real-world touchstone" (Angel 52) and saviour (Kavadlo 8).

Regardless of Marla's ontological status, Joe's self-help groups turn out be an extraordinarily precarious form of ego therapy. For one thing, in spite of the cathartic intimacy he is able to experience with his fellow attendees, he slowly begins to recognize that the groups engage in a new age disavowal of the fragmentary life of the body:

> Eyes closed, we imagined our pain as a ball of white healing light floating around our feet and rising to our knees, our waist, our chest. Our

> chakras opening. The heart chakra, the head chakra. Chloe talked us into caves where we met our power animal. Mine was a penguin.
>
> Ice covered the floor of the cave, and the penguin said slide. Without any effort, we slide through tunnels and galleries.
>
> Then it was time to hug. . . . This was therapeutic physical contact, Chloe said.
>
> (20)

Chloe's brand of therapy effects the phantasmal relocation of the spirit, the erasure of the mortal body, and the disavowal of its limits. As such, this new age fantasy system adds another layer of dissimulation to Joe's already deracinated experience. The disassembly of his body into chakras and relocation of his soul within a frictionless, painless metaphysical milieu re-inscribes him within the eviscerating neoliberal order and compounds as many of Joe's problems as it purports to dissolve.

The limitations of new age self-help are evident from the beginning. Joe's first experience of catharsis in these groups is in Remaining Men Together. In a gender-bending embrace with Bob (whose large breasts and loving embrace figure him as an ersatz mother within what is supposed to be a strictly homosocial community), he experiences a strange admixture of comfort and discomfort:

> Big Bob was a juicer, he said. All those salad days on Dianabol and then the racehorse steroid, Wistrol. His own gym, Big Bob owned a gym. He'd been married three times. He'd done product endorsements, and had I seen him on television, ever? The whole how-to-program about expanding your chest was practically his invention.
>
> Strangers with this kind of honesty make me go a big rubbery one, if you know what I mean.
>
> Bob didn't know. Maybe only one of his huevos had ever descended, and he knew this was a risk factor. Bob told me about post-operative hormone therapy.
>
> A lot of bodybuilders shooting too much testosterone would get what they called bitch tits.
>
> I had to ask what Bob meant by huevos.
>
> Huevos, Bob said. Gonads. Nuts. Jewels. Testes. Balls. In Mexico, where you buy your steroids, they call them "eggs."
>
> (21)

In "Violence, Space, Fragmenting Consciousness," James Giles observes that Bob, who has had his cancerous testicles removed before meeting Joe at Remaining Men Together, "functions as an ironic embodiment of the narrator's own fear of emasculation" (31). But Bob figures as much more than an embodiment of Joe's concerns about remaining a normative man.

His account of his own trajectory mirrors and figures as a metonym for Joe's entire itinerary. Seduced by idealized media images of the "beautiful stock body" (48), Bob has pursued this commodified hypermasculine ideal with dogged determination and the aid of a powerful pharmacopeia. However, the hypermasculating steroids and hormones have ruined his health, dashed his family against the rocks, effeminized him with "bitch tits," and, ultimately, induced semi-castration; even the putative biological loci of his manhood – his testicles – are wounded, regendered, re-ethnicized, and even assigned a different species as "huevos." Bob's slavish efforts to achieve the masculine ideal have culminated in perverse effeminization, indexing the seeming impossibility of normatively Remaining Men Together.

Après-Coup: Bodies in Splices

For Joe, Marla's feminine incursions and Bob's effeminization betoken the impossibility of properly remasculating and authentically rejoining humanity through support groups. Joe – or, rather, his unconscious – is left with no choice but to devise a new strategy to re-inflate his "big rubbery one." It is at this moment, in the midst of this crisis of masculine integrity, that he first encounters his alter ego, Tyler Durden.

When Tyler first enters the picture, he has two primary jobs. He is a banquet waiter at a fancy downtown hotel and a film projectionist. In both occupations, he engages in small-scale guerrilla vandalism. As a waiter, he routinely engages in "dinner party sabot[age]" (81), sticking his erect penis in, urinating in, and flatulating on banquet food before it is served to eminent guests like "the Empire State Lawyers" (80). As a projectionist, Tyler's favourite pastime is splicing pornographic images of penises into mainstream films. As a paragon of exuberant, enfranchised masculinity, Tyler asserts his tumescent manhood everywhere, including the big screen:

> Tyler spliced a penis into everything after that. Usually, close-ups . . . four stories tall and twitching with blood pressure as Cinderella danced with her Prince Charming and people watched. . . . People ate and drank, but the evening wasn't the same. People feel sick or start to cry and don't know why.
>
> (31)

In "A Generation of Men Without History," Krister Friday asserts that Tyler's "pornographic intrusion[s]" (Friday 3) "encapsulat[e] *Fight Club*'s narrative logic and its complex imaginative imbrication of identity and historical self-consciousness. . . . [W]hat Tyler inserts is a single, subliminal frame that represents a moment of masculine prowess" (Friday 1). Looking to Sally Robinson's gender-theoretical work on white masculinity, Friday underscores the role of a master narrative of "white male decline prevalent in post-sixties, white-male American fiction" (Robinson 2; qtd. in Friday 7): "Robinson argues that such narratives construct a notion of male victimization and its related symptomology [sic] as redress for a perceived political and social emasculation" (Friday 7). These narratives function as "a way of compensating for a sense of disempowerment created by a contemporary culture in which the white male no longer occupies a central, unchallenged normative position" (7). Friday observes that this perception of emasculation sets in motion a "compensatory trajectory" (Friday 7) of masculine reassertion, coding itself "in terms of the scandalous and the prohibited" (Friday 7). By embarking on this compensatory arc, Joe seeks to overcome this perceived crisis of white masculinity "through a redemptive recovery of male prowess" (Friday 12). But he does so under castrating conditions whereby "any male identity that exists is simultaneously on the brink of extinction, not emergence" (Friday 12).

As with Bob's hormonal therapy, Durden's penis splices serve as an even more explicitly medial trope for the fraught effort to reassert atavistic masculinity under the symbolically castrated, hypermediated conditions of media modernity. These detached and wounded penises are, Cynthia Kuhn claims, just a few of many organs without bodies circulating through the text: "in *Fight Club*, fragmented bodies constantly serve as literal reminders and as metaphorical responses to the complexities of negotiating cultural expectations" (Kuhn 39). Kuhn cites Project Mayhem's castration threats, Marla's dildo, and the narrator's references to himself as individual body parts all as instances of bodily disintegration,

> reflect[ing] his psychic disintegration, crossing from biological – 'I am totally Joe's Gallbladder' . . . – to emotive territory: 'I am Joe's Boiling Point' . . . . In this latter move, sentiment appears to be unsuitable in 'masculine' terms unless splintered and proffered in a sarcastic way.
> (Kuhn 40)

Tyler inserts the spliced penises, which Kuhn refers to as "cinematic vivisections" (Kuhn 39), to reassert his masculinity and " 'giv[e] the finger' to mainstream consumerist society" (Giles 28). Nevertheless, the overriding diegetic logic of these cinematic surgeries only further fragments Joe as he struggles, Humpty-Dumpty-like, to put himself back together again. Joe is, in effect, the ultimate object of his countless medial "vivisections."

Remanning *Big Rubbery Men*

Slavoj Žižek views *Fight Club* as a staging ground of different interpenetrating categories of violence. In *Violence: Six Sideways Reflections*, he proposes a political–psychoanalytic triangle of violence that sheds light on Joe's compensatory arc by categorizing violence under three inter-oriented rubrics.

The first and most obvious is "subjective violence," obtrusively violent acts "performed by a clearly identifiable agent" (*Violence* 1). The second is "symbolic violence," the "social domination" that emerges out of "the imposition of a certain universe of meaning" (*Violence* 2) on the world. The final category is "systemic violence," which he characterizes as the pernicious operation of "virtual capitalism" (*Violence* 13), whose often invisible speculative operations callously run roughshod over people, environments, and economies.

In the age of digital biopolitics, the click of a mouse button in a placid-seeming Manhattan office can, in the blink of an eye, put an entire town out of work across the globe or cancel an automobile recall that could have saved thousands of lives. Systemic violence is often conveniently invisible to those who are not directly impacted by it. This is because it operates in collaboration with symbolic violence, the violence of language and culture, qua "parasitic symbolic machine[ry]" (*Parallax* 121), to "posit meaning while concealing the meaningless machinery of its own linguistic positing" (Edelman 104). At its most sinister, "objective violence," constituted by the complex interplay of systemic and symbolic violence, manifests itself in the ideology of frictionless capitalism, a conceit that cynically obscures the viciousness of neoliberalism by conjuring an idealized world of virtualized, disembodied transactions without deleterious impacts on laborers, the environment, or the economy at large. Far from being the exception to the rule in an otherwise tranquil world, objective violence permeates all symbolic codifications and social transactions, regardless of how subjectively peaceful they may seem. In other words, the fantasy of a world without violence, or even friction, is ideology at its purest. Our habituation to the displacement and concealment of systemic and symbolic violence impels us to sensationalize subjective violence to the extent that we do.

On this matter of divergent phenomenologies of violence, Žižek cites Bertolt Brecht's provocation:

> What is the robbery of a bank compared to the founding of a bank? In other words, what is the robbery that violates the law compared to the robbery that takes place within the confines of the law? One is tempted to propose a new variation of this motto: what is committing an act of terror to a state power waging war on terror?
>
> (Violence 117)

Accordingly, Žižek contends that the putatively tranquil occupation of contemporary office work is a primary site of this dialectic, as exemplified by the volatile interplay of all three modalities of violence cutting into Joe's life. In Tyler's fight club, Joe finds a seemingly potent corrective to the symbolic violence of his castrating filing-cabinet universe. Fight club is, in a sense, the sublation of his subjectively peaceful but objectively violent form of life.

It is his first deliberate project to negate his own disavowal of violence by aggressively embracing it. With the collapse of the support groups' viability as therapeutic vehicles to help him "feel alive," he fabricates *a new lease on life* through the lived experience of fight club.[4]

Like the therapy groups, fight club seizes upon embodiment in the form of "therapeutic physical contact" in order to connect with other men and escape from his moribund lifestyle. But, unlike the support groups, fight club rejects tranquil new age fantasies of ego-unity and escape from the mortal body. Instead, it embraces the emancipatory ego-shattering potentials of violence and pain:

> You aren't alive anywhere like you're alive at fight club. When it's you and one other guy under that one light in the middle of all those watching. Fight club isn't about winning or losing fights. Fight club isn't about words. You see a guy come to fight club for the first time, and his ass is a loaf of white bread. You see this same guy here six months later, and he looks carved out of wood. This guy trusts himself to handle anything. There's grunting and noise at fight club like at the gym, but fight club isn't about looking good. There's hysterical shouting in tongues like at church, and when you wake up Sunday . . . you feel saved.
>
> (51)

In contradistinction to the arc of castrated masculinity exemplified by the likes of Bob, Durden's fight club offers a therapeutic, seemingly unmediated experience of rugged masculinity through spiritualized combat.

Again, on the topic of fight club's rugged immediacy as a corrective to the culture industry's categorical imperatives, Joe notes,

> I don't want to die without a few scars. . . . It's nothing anymore to have a beautiful stock body. You see those cars that are completely stock cherry, right out of a dealer's showroom in 1955, I always think what a waste. . . . It used to be enough that when I came home angry and knowing that my life wasn't toeing my five-year plan, I could clean my condominium or detail my car. Someday I'd be dead without a scar and there would be a really nice condo and car. Really, really nice, until the dust settled or the next owner. Nothing is static. Even the Mona Lisa is falling apart. Since fight club, I can wiggle half the teeth in my jaw. Maybe self-improvement isn't the answer.
>
> Tyler never knew his father.
>
> Maybe self-destruction is the answer.
>
> (48–49)

Rejecting egoic unity and the cultural commodification of the male "stock body," Durden's approach to life embraces friction, fragmentation, and pain, which it "sublate[s] into affirmative joy" (Diken and Laustsen 7). Nevertheless, the fact that Joe frames fight club as transforming the (presumably white) "loaf of bread" and cherry "stock body" into something "carved out of wood" should give the critical reader pause, as this is not the first wood to go under the knife in this text.

Immediacy and Its Discontents

The notion of men "carved out of wood" also seems to allude to Joe's first meeting with Tyler, whom he discovered gathering driftwood on the beach to build a rarefied sundial, of sorts, that projected a shadowy hand onto the sand at precisely 4:30 pm. This new age exercise in evanescence, and the first of Tyler's medial vivisections, serves as a Dionysian counterpoint to Joe's life-long Apollonian project of fabricating his self-image and making himself whole through the right purchases. The wooden construction, which the sun fleetingly mediates into a human hand and then a kind of inhuman "Nosferatu" hand, in turn invokes the scene at the very opening of the novel (also not represented in the film) in which Tyler tells Joe they'll be the stuff of legend and live forever, to which Joe responds, "you're thinking of vampires" (12). Thus, this prehensile "organ without a body" would seem to serve as a synecdoche for the monstrous economy within which Joe finds himself as he struggles to occupy a viable subject position that makes him feel immediate, manly, and alive. Insofar as fight club fashions men into aggressively self-asserting phalluses that are immune to the commodifying, effeminizing, dehumanizing tendencies of late twentieth-century American culture, it also re-inscribes their precarious "wood" within an ever-unfurling and castrating socio-symbolic matrix.

When fight club is still in its infancy, Joe would like to believe that it is an immediate panacea to the *pharmakon* of passively consumed hypermediated violence:

> Fight club is not football on television. You aren't watching a bunch of men you don't know halfway around the world beating on each other live by satellite with a two-minute delay, commercials pitching beer every ten minutes, and a pause now for station identification. After you've been to fight club, watching football on television is watching pornography when you could be having great sex.
>
> (50)

As with all of Joe's utterances, his discourse merits close reading. For one thing, the analogy with heteronormative sex betrays his own homoerotic (and therefore effeminized, according to the dominant discourse) investment in fight club. Moreover, it is Joe who opts to consume and create pornography when he "could be having great sex" (with Marla), a traditionally heteronormative undertaking so unpalatable that he can only mediate it through Tyler.

Whether he realizes it or not, his own narrative account of fight club's inherent mediality flies in the face of any pretences of immediacy or normative manliness:

> Like every guy on his first night in fight club, I breathed in and swung my fist in a roundhouse at Tyler's jaw like in every cowboy movie we'd ever seen, and me, my fist connected with the side of Tyler's neck.
>
> Shit, I said, that didn't count. I want to try it again.
>
> Tyler said, "Yeah it counted," and hit me, straight on, pow, just like a cartoon boxing glove on a spring on Saturday morning cartoons, right in the middle of my chest and I fell back against a car. We both stood there, Tyler rubbing the side of his neck and me holding a hand on my chest, both of us knowing we'd gotten somewhere we'd never been and like the cat and mouse in cartoons, we were still alive and wanted to see how far we could take this thing and still be alive. . . .
>
> I said, hit me again.
>
> Tyler said, "No, you hit me."
>
> So I hit him. . . . What happened next and after that didn't happen in words.
>
> (53)

Even in the process of lionizing fight club for its pre-symbolic immediacy, Joe divulges that his strong, silent enactment of embodied masculinity is a recrudescence of the same infantile, disembodied media diet that has landed him here in the first place. It seems his vigilant efforts to re-inscribe his phallus into the scene are always going to be purloined and spliced into even more simulacrally castrating cartoon productions.

Cynthia Kuhn notes that fight clubbers' flailing attempts to remasculate are destined to fall flat from the outset. Their efforts to "become 'men' are hindered by taking cues from cultural representations of 'masculinity' rather than from an intimate relationship with a father figure" (Kuhn 38). She adds, "they have been left to deal with the consequences of paternal sin – i.e., abandonment – and feeling lost in the figurative ancestral curse" (Kuhn 38). Indeed, the spectral absent father figure is very much in the crosshairs of Tyler's project: "most guys are at fight club because of something they're too scared to fight. After a few fights, you're afraid a lot less" (54). When Joe asks Tyler what he is fighting against, "Tyler said, his father" (53). Once again, in spite of the illusion of immediacy that it fosters, fight club proves itself to be deracinatingly mediated. As a venue for misdirected aggression, fight club is archetypical "acting out" in that it serves as a kind of confrontational simulation, a testing ground for and displacement of a thoroughly Oedipal paternal confrontation. The real target of fight club is the absent law-creating father, but this confrontation can never take place in reality. The primal horde is left without a proper object and must slavishly await instructions as to where to direct its aggression.

Purloined Polemics

As fight club engulfs every aspect of his life, Joe directs more and more hostility towards his workplace and the capitalist system of domination that it conducts. In addition to proudly brandishing his combat wounds at the office, he authors and distributes dissident missives:

> The hole punched through my cheek doesn't ever heal. I'm going to work, and my punched-out eye sockets are two swollen up black bagels around the little piss holes I have to see through. Until today, it really pissed me off that I'd become this totally centered Zen Master and nobody had noticed. Still, I'm doing the little FAX thing. I write little HAIKU things and FAX them around to everyone. When I pass people in the hall at work, I get totally ZEN right in everyone's hostile little FACE.
>
> (63)

His antagonistic behaviour towards his co-workers and employer is arguably a misplaced pugnacious response to the violence of wage slavery and its corrosive impact on his life. It is noteworthy that this confrontation takes the form of a replica – through the medium of the fax machine – of the Buddhist themes Joe encounters in his support group sessions. But in its reconstituted form, Joe's new age wisdom, far from concealing or mitigating the frictions of capitalism, emanates out of a self-styled "Zen" mastery that enables him to wield and amplify aggression.

One of Joe's fax haikus reads like a contemporary poetic variant on Hegel's master–slave dialectic: "Worker bees can leave/Even drones can fly away/The queen is their slave" (63). Another, which he composes in his head in response to his boss' questions about the blood on his face, is a ruminative piece about work/life balance: "Without just one nest/A bird can call the world home/Life is your career" (64). While the support group's new age fantasy system was meant to be a soothing ego balm to render the difficult life of wage slavery more tolerable, Joe's newfound enlightenment (however sardonic) is a call to insurrection against the hegemony of a sick late-capitalist order. But it is by no means clear who the proper recipients of his messages are. The poems could be intended for his own meditative edification, his co-workers, and/or his employer. But given that these faxes are, like the photocopies circulating through the office, emblematic of a simulacral fantasmatic economy, he may well be hallucinating everything about this episode. Regardless, this clarion call to rebel against a perversely hostile system gestures toward the next metamorphosis of fight club into the terroristic Project Mayhem.

Commenting on the spread of fight club and its connection to his workplace, Joe observes that at meetings and conferences he encounters fellow office workers

> with broken noses spreading out like an eggplant under the edges of bandages or they have a couple stitches under an eye or a jaw wired shut. These are the quiet young men who listen until it's time to decide.
>
> (54)

In response to these men's battle scars, Joe's boss quips that "there are fewer and fewer gentlemen in business and more thugs" (54). According to Giles, such "images of badly mutilated young men at business conferences constitute an early clue of the fundamental unreality of fight club. Obviously, no corporation would retain such employees, much less send them to high-level conferences" (Giles 36). There is a much-overlooked irony to the assertion that there are "fewer and fewer gentlemen in business." As Giles frames the matter,

> the boss, off course, is one of the individuals who decide not to issue recalls, even when the lives of consumers are endangered. He, like those above him on the corporate ladder, is himself a dangerous thug, no matter the decency of his public appearance.
>
> (Giles 36)

Fight club, then, renders visible Joe's dawning awareness of his corporation's perpetration of far-reaching objective violence on both others and himself. And, once again, though he attempts to mobilize what Žižek calls "subjective violence" in the direction of agency and authenticity, his bruises bespeak the traumatic spiritual beatings that he has received by way of his collusion in this corporate necropolitical matrix.

Partial Abjects: Repetition With a Vas Deferens

According to Žižek, Joe's masochistic confrontation with his boss takes him one step closer to an uncanny form of agency:

> To blackmail his boss . . . the hero throws himself around the man's office, beating himself bloody. . . . In front of his embarrassed boss, the narrator thus enacts upon himself the boss' aggression toward him. . . . The self-beating begins with the hero's hand acquiring a life of its own, escaping the hero's control – in short, turning into a partial object, or, to put it in Deleuze's terms, into *an organ without a body* (the obverse

> of the *body without organs*). This provides the key to the double with whom . . . the hero is fighting. His double, the hero's Ideal-Ego, a spectral/invisible hallucinatory entity – not simply external to the hero. Its efficacy is inscribed within the hero's body itself as the autonomization of one of its organs. . . . The hand acting on its own is the drive ignoring the dialectic of the subject's desire: drive is fundamentally the insistence of an undead "organ without a body," standing, like Lacan's *lamella*, for that which the subject had to lose in order to subjectivize itself in the symbolic space of the sexual difference.
>
> (*Organs* 173–174)

Žižek's analysis locates many of the ironic coordinates of the scene: Joe deliberately dissembles that his boss is beating him up by simultaneously occupying the roles of beater and beaten; according to Žižek, this is a fundamentally masochistic revolutionary gesture. By choreographing the scene and assuming both roles, he transitions from being an unreflective instrument of the callous capitalist system to an agentive usurper of its monopoly on the legitimate use of violence.

Žižek frames Joe's inversion as a potentially emancipatory act because it unveils the vicious logic subtending the seemingly placid workplace:

> So when [Joe] beats himself up in front of his boss, his message to the boss is: "I know you want to beat me, but you see, your desire to beat me is also my desire, so if you were to beat me, you would be fulfilling the role of the servant of my perverse masochistic desire. But you're too much of a coward to act out your desire, so I'll do it for you – here it is, you've got what you really wanted. Why are you so embarrassed? Aren't you ready to accept it?" The gap between fantasy and reality is crucial here: the boss, of course, would never actually have beaten [Joe] up, he was merely fantasizing about doing it, and the painful effect of [Joe's] self-beating hinges on the very fact that he stages the content of the secret fantasy his boss would never be able to actualize.
>
> (*Revolution* 251)

Joe's subversive gesture begins with his perverse expropriation of the boss' role in a system that wields control over of him. He begins the episode with a phone call to the city desk of a local newspaper to confess, in front of his employer, to the disgusting guerrilla vandalism that he has been engaging in at the hotel; he claims to have "committed a terrible crime against humanity as part of a political protest . . . over the exploitation of workers in the service industry" (115). By confessing to his "protest" and punching himself, he transfigures the systemic violence to which he has been submitted into "subjective" (i.e., visible) violence and renders its viciousness legible.

Moreover, Joe's masochistic choreography, according to Žižek's reading, reaveals that, "even on a purely formal level, . . . the master is superfluous." Ventriloquizing Joe, he continues, "'Who needs you to terrorize me? I can do it myself!' So it is only through [self-inflicted violence] that one becomes free: the true goal . . . is to beat out that in me which attaches me to the master" (Revolution 252).

While fight club's experiment in channelling aggression can be understood as a hapless venue for "acting out" against the absent father, Žižek characterizes Joe's transition towards protest as a "passage to the act" bordering on an authentic act of liberation. This claim merits closer analysis because it is an important one. Lacanian psychoanalysis frames acting out as

> a ciphered message which the subject addresses to an Other, although the subject himself is neither conscious of the content of this message nor even aware that his actions express a message. It is the Other who is entrusted with deciphering the message; yet it is impossible for him to do so.
>
> (Evans 3)

A passage to the act, on the other hand, is an often psychotic "flight from the Other into the dimension of the real. The passage to the act is thus an exit from the symbolic network, a dissolution of the social bond" (Evans 140). Unlike acting out, a passage to the act is "not a message addressed to anyone, since symbolisation ha[s] become impossible" (Evans 140). While Joe does ultimately migrate from misdirected messages to his absent father to a near-suicidal exit from the stage of the play, he also, according to Žižek's reading, takes a necessary step in the direction of seizing power from his oppressive employer in a manner that anticipates twenty-first century activist efforts to occupy the occupier. But the status of this step remains ambiguous.

Focusing on the arc of David Fincher's film adaptation, Žižek writes,

> Paradoxically, such a staging is the first act of liberation. By means of it, the servant's masochist libidinal attachment to his master is brought to the daylight, and the servant thus acquires a minimal distance toward it. Already at a purely formal level, the fact of beating up oneself renders clear the simple fact that the master is superfluous: "Who needs you for terrorizing me? I can do it myself!" It is thus only through first beating up (hitting) oneself that one becomes free: The true goal of this beating is to beat out that which in me attaches me to the master. When, toward the end, [Joe] shoots at himself (surviving the shot, effectively killing only "Tyler in himself," his double), he thereby also liberates himself from the dual mirror-relationship of beating. In this culmination of self-aggression, its logic cancels itself, [he] will no longer have

> to beat himself – now he will be able to beat the true enemy (the system).
>
> ("The Violence of the Fantasy" 286)

Of course, it bears repeating that Joe is able to galvanize this heroic agency at the end of David Fincher's film, but the ending of Palahniuk's novel is much more ambiguous. The film adaptation ends with Joe murdering Tyler and nearly killing himself in order to save Marla and perhaps the world. With Tyler's demise, Joe and Marla stand alone, bearing witness to the decimation of the office towers that house the businesses responsible for the oppression of the underclasses. In contrast, Palahniuk's novel ends with Joe in a mental hospital, where, it turns out, he has likely hallucinated the entire ordeal, including not only Tyler Durden but also Marla Singer and even the annihilation of the Parker Morris Building.

But there is another flaw in Žižek's reading as it applies to the representation of emancipatory violence in the novel. Joe's staged altercation with his boss ends ambiguously. He does not merely assume of the boss' position of mastery; a monstrous agency bubbles to the surface and thwarts Joe's aspiration to assert control over the scene:

> I punch myself again, again. It just looks good, all the blood, but I throw myself back against the wall to make a terrible noise and break the painting that hangs there. The broken glass and frame and the painting of flowers and blood go to the floor with me clowning around. . . . Blood gets on the carpet and I reach up and grip *monster handprints* of blood on the edge of the hotel manager's desk and say, please, help me. . . . Please don't hit me, again. I slip back to the floor and crawl my blood across the carpet. . . . *The monster drags itself* across the lovely bouquets and garlands of the Oriental carpet. . . . And this is how Tyler was free to start a fight club every night of the week. . . . *The monster hooks its bloody claw* in the waistband of the manager's pants, and pulls itself up to clutch the white starched shirt, and I wrap my bloody hands around the manager's smooth wrists.
>
> (116–117; my emphases)

Joe's effort to violently assert his own masculine agency in this inescapably mediatized space, in turn, renders his hand into something monstrous, the *lamella* of a demonic power that violently occupies his subjectivity and transfigures fight club into Project Mayhem. "Violent excess," writes Giles, "rather than controlling reason is the defining ingredient of . . . fight club. Such devotion to excess negates any possibility that the narrator will control the fantasy; in fact, as the novel progresses, it increasingly controls him" (Giles 35). Žižek is astute to characterize Joe's behaviour as bordering on an authentic political act that empowers him to confront his boss and the pernicious socio-symbolic order that he represents. But his analysis also overlooks the extent to which Joe's unwieldly franchise takes on an undead life of its own as the project metastasizes.

Reign of Error

In its final metamorphosis, fight club, avers Giles, "extends beyond the promotion of simple fighting and assumes a broader mission," Project Mayhem, the perpetration of more far-reaching acts of terror, especially on large corporations. "Project Mayhem operates according to a set of rules, promulgated of course by Tyler Durden, that mimic those of fight club itself" (Giles 36). "The first rule about Project Mayhem," announces Durden, "is that you don't ask questions about Project Mayhem" (119). And, like the corporate world, Project Mayhem operates through committees: "That Project Mayhem is modeled on the corporate world demonstrates that the narrator has been so co-opted by that world that, ironically, he does not resist it in his fantasy of rebellion" (Giles 36). The description of Project Mayhem committees as "support groups. Sort of" (119) contains "an important clue" (Giles 36) about the recursive logic of the narrative.

It therefore makes sense to interpret Project Mayhem as a quasi-Hegelian stage of Joe's dissident metamorphosis. Diken and Laustsen observe that, in Project Mayhem, "pain is sublated into terror. . . . To cure one's pain one needs to demolish the system that creates it" (Diken and Laustsen 7).

However, when the violence is directed outwards, it becomes increasingly difficult to "distinguish between fascism and benevolent terror" in the service of a greater cause. "The difference," Diken and Laustsen contend, "is the subject serving as the agent of violence" (Diken and Laustsen 7). This leads them to ask, "Does the subject heroically accept its role as a vanishing mediator? Does the revolutionary act transform the subject? Or, does it lay the ground for a regime of terror sustained by an unchanged subject?" (Diken and Laustsen 7-8).

In spite of Tyler's occasional anti-capitalist oratory, Project Mayhem would seem to recapitulate the malevolent (violent, fascistic, homogenizing) tendencies of the dominant order against which it is presumably meant to be an insurgency. As such, it functions as a sort of negation of the original negation (i.e., fight club) of Joe's dehumanized, emasculated life. Thus, despite Tyler's polemics against corporatism and consumerism, he is still possessed by their spirit:

> I wanted to destroy everything beautiful I'd never have. . . . Open the dump valves on supertankers and uncap offshore oil wells. I wanted to kill all the fish I couldn't afford to eat, and smother the French beaches I'd never see. . . .

> I wanted the whole world to hit bottom.
>
> . . . I really wanted to put a bullet between the eyes of every endangered panda that wouldn't screw to save its species and every whale or dolphin that gave up and ran itself aground.
>
> Don't think of this as extinction. Think of this as downsizing.
>
> (123–124)

This impulse, claims Kavadlo, amounts to the "apolitical destruction of an apathetic world, a way for the powerless to fantasize about spiting nature" (Kavadlo 11). "The language," Kavadlo continues, "is still that of consumption – seeing fish as edible commodity, for example. He still employs the same consumerist thinking, only with the sentiments reversed: the obsession with acquisition has turned into a desire for its removal" (Kavadlo 11). In contrast to, say, the contemporary Idle No More movement, which sought to re-occupy the colonial occupier by short-circuiting the necropolitical devaluation of life and death, Tyler embraces a new twist on systemic violence. Joe's impetus to be a docile employee has morphed into a drive to usurp the "downsizing" boss and ruthlessly occupy the position of Master.

God's Media Children

Joe's occupational universe and its relationship to the Law of the Father figure prominently in Project Mayhem. As this next stage begins to unfurl, the mechanic whom Joe encounters at the paper street house recites some "Tyler Durden dogma" (141):

> What you have to understand is your father was your model for God. . . . If you're male and you're Christian and living in America, your father is your model for God. And if you never know your father, if your father bails out or dies or is never at home, what do you believe about God? . . . What you end up doing . . . is you spend your life searching for a father and God. . . . Burn the Louvre . . . and wipe your ass with the Mona Lisa. This way at least, God would know our names. . . . As long as you're at fight club, you're not how much money you've got in the bank. You're not your job. You're not your family, and you're not who you tell yourself. . . . You're not your name.
>
> (141–143)

Tyler's screed against the Name of the Father induces in Joe a sense of déjà-vu as he surmises that it was "scrawled on bits of paper while [he] was asleep and given to [him] to type and photocopy at work. . . . [He has] read it all. Even [his] boss has probably read it all" (141). Recalling the mantra, Joe adds "We are God's middle children, according to Tyler Durden, with no special place in history and no special attention" (141). Tyler's aspiration to usurp the absolute paternal signifier (which is actually a flickering oscillation between God, his flesh-and-blood father, history, and his boss) is not as straightforward as he would have his recruits believe. If the white, middle-class, Christian male recruits are rechristened as anonymous "space monkeys," then their individual names will never accrue the personal or historical significance that they strive after. They are, rather, experimental fodder for a great dissident experiment whose ultimate outcome will be wildly chaotic. What's more, the ambition to have "God . . . know [their] names" suggests that whatever stage in the master–slave dialectic they manage to reach, they will always operate under the panoptical scrutiny of an imagined paternal agency whose unassailable structural function is to subordinate their fulminations to its authority.

The mechanic continues with a panegyric that is "pure Tyler Durden":

> I see the strongest and the smartest men who have ever lived . . . and these men are pumping gas and waiting tables. If we could put these men in training camps and finish raising them. All a gun does is focus an explosion in one direction.
>
> You have a class of young strong men and women, and they want to give their lives to something. Advertising has these people chasing cars and clothes they don't need. Generations have been working in jobs they hate, just so they can buy what they don't really need. We don't have a great war in our generation, or a great depression, but we do, we have a great war of the spirit. We have a great revolution against the culture. The great depression is our lives. We have a spiritual depression. We have to show these men and women freedom by enslaving them, and show them courage by frightening them. Napoleon bragged that he could train men to sacrifice their lives for a scrap of ribbon. Imagine, when we call a strike and everyone refuses to work until we redistribute the wealth of the world. Imagine hunting elk through the damp canyon forests around the ruins of Rockefeller Center.
>
> (149–150)

The narrative logic of this passage is, by now, clear. Durden devised Project Mayhem as a remedy to the crippling malaise of modern masculinity. By attacking and dismantling the dominant order, he seeks to reassert a new form of tyranny, with Tyler occupying the castrating Napoleonic position hitherto held by the hegemonic advertising industry. And as the nature of the *Unbehagen* continues to morph, Joe's insomnia, which has given way to an array of fake illnesses, now manifests itself as a "depression." Due to this quasi-Jamesonian "waning of affect," on account of the lack of grand militarist narratives to marshal and unify the generation's *jouissance*, Tyler has emerged to fill the void with Project Mayhem. In the middle of an epideictic lecture about how Project Mayhem is "going to save the world [by forcing] humanity to go dormant long enough for the Earth to recover," Tyler tips his hand as to its libidinal underpinnings: "'You justify anarchy,' Tyler says. 'You figure it out.'" (125).

Passion for the Reel

In accordance with the medial logic of *Fight Club*, Joe imagines the demolition of the Parker Morris-Building as a succession of film frames:

> The demolition team will hit the primary charge in maybe eight minutes. The primary charge will blow the base charge, the foundation columns will crumble, and the photo series of the Parker-Morris Building will go into all the History books. The five-picture time lapse series. Here the building's standing. Second picture, the building will be at an eighty-degree angle. Then a seventy-degree angle. The building's at a forty-five-degree-angle in the fourth picture when the skeleton starts to give and the tower gets a slight arch to it. The last shot, the tower, all one hundred and ninety-one floors, will slam down on the national museum which is Tyler's real target.
>
> (14)

That the detonation will go into "all the History books" flies in the face of Project Mayhem's goal to annihilate "every scrap of history" (12). No matter how he targets the Big Other, it will reconstitute itself as a spectral agency. Even if the museum is destroyed, Durden will never succeed at liquidating the structural role of the God's–eye view. The chaos would necessarily be re-inscribed within the virtual archive, and the space monkeys' Oedipal revolt will always fall short of the pantheon of cosmic significance.

These frames gesture towards the "pornographic intrusions" at the beginning of the novel:

> A single frame in a movie is on the screen for one-sixtieth of a second. Divide a second into sixty equal parts. That's how long the erection is. Towering four stories tall over the popcorn auditorium, slippery red and terrible, and no one sees it.
>
> (30)

The "towering" multi-story erection frame that Tyler splices into the children's film presages the culmination of the dialectic in Project Mayhem's demolition of the Parker-Morris Building and the whole narrative universe of *Fight Club* is unmoored from any pretence of a God's–eye view or metahistorical position from which all of the variables of the situation cohere in such a way that they can be mastered or rendered intelligible. The reader and Joe converge on the insight that there is always another subliminal agency, another "frame of reference," whose interventions cannot be accounted for, even by the most comprehensive "liability formula."

Breaking the First Rule of Fight Club

Marshall McLuhan famously believed that there is a particular category of art that operates as an "early warning system" capable of "anticipat[ing] future social and technological developments" as well as their "psychic and social consequences" (McLuhan xi). Narrative universes like *Fight Club* harbour the potential to provide what McLuhan viewed as "indispensable perceptual training" (xi) that can aid readers in momentarily snapping out of the somnambulistic stupor induced by our absolute immersion in a psychotropic infotainment environment.

Although he is best remembered for his celebration of the eruption of media modernity, McLuhan's enthusiasm was far from untempered. He believed that artistic and philosophical short-circuits of our mesmeric media bubbles hold out the fragile hope of guiding humanity towards a more mature form of media literacy. By developing a measure of critical distance from its electrified atmospheres, humanity could cultivate an ever-evolving political-mediatic compass with which to chart "an even course toward permanent goals, even amidst the most disrupting innovations" (xi).

It is unfortunate that *Fight Club* occupies such a stigmatized, hemmed-in place in the contemporary American imaginary. This circumscription is in no small part a consequence of the deep integration of the lineaments of David Fincher's film adaptation into a pop-cultural environment that flattens out complexity and homogenizes nuance. Still, the pervasive caricaturization of *Fight Club* is more than a little ironic. For those who still take on the task of reading and talking about it, Palahniuk's novel continues to resonate as a potent allegory of the very same undertows of media modernity to which it has largely succumbed.

A superficial reading of *Fight Club* that dwells on Durden's terroristic itinerary may even lead some to assume that the novel is a wholesale critique of anti-capitalist activism and the supposed "snowflakes" that promulgate it.[5] The novel certainly does not readily lend itself to such assumptions. As Žižek makes clear, "the first lesson of *Fight Club* is . . . that one cannot pass directly from capitalist to revolutionary subjectivity" ("The Violence of the Fantasy" 285). Indeed, Joe's drive to conduct his successive dissident projects through the very fascistic neoliberal coordinates they are meant to overthrow betokens his umbilicus to a capitalist subjectivity and moribund patriarchal order. This begets questions about how the insights gleaned from the era's early warning systems can be mobilized in the direction of vibrant revolutionary subjectivity.

"Not Me. Us": Manufacturing the Right Kind of Desire

In the wake of 9/11, the psychotic "War on Terror," the 2007 economic crisis, and the Covid-19 pandemic, few honest observers would characterize the contemporary world as a frictionless disembodied milieu in spite of frequent assertions to the contrary emanating out of the mindfulness industry. *Fight Club* depicts Joe's psychotic unravelling in relation to a caustic neoliberal machine that persuades slavish consumers that they are unique snowflakes while rendering life, subjectivity, and community into meaningless, interchangeable commodities. It should come as no surprise that Durden's increasingly cynical responses to the violence internalized by Joe conduct and reconfigure that same violence in a sinister and chaotic fashion. But Durden's nihilistic kamikaze mission is not the only possible trajectory out of his important insights into the obscene violence of the American project at the end of the twentieth century; nor, for that matter, is Joe's psychotic meltdown.

Modifying and elaborating on Žižek's theorization of revolutionary subjectivity, Jodi Dean distinguishes "inward-turning" drive-based "repetitive circuits," such as Joe's recursive metamorphoses, from what she refers to as a "collective desire for collectivity." "Desire," she claims "doesn't turn inward; it looks outward, toward the horizon." Such an outward-turning politics of desire "break[s] out of the trap of reflexivity, [by] installing a gap . . . a rupture of the circuit that lets us look outwards" ("Admitting"). For Dean, this short-circuit emerges out of a subtle balance between competent leadership and the communal understanding that vibrant political collectives "bring together people with different skills, experience, and knowledge" ("Admitting") to create a better world.

Fight Club would seem to lend itself to the conservative critique that contemporary protest movements like Occupy Wall Street are, at best, destined to collapse in on themselves and, at worst, likely to flip over into free-floating terror. While critics of Occupy Wall Street are quick to underscore its lack of coherent agenda and political gravity (and some of these critiques are, indeed, justified), the movement has sent out ripples that conjure a compelling contrast to fight club's thanatotic political itinerary. In a turn that would have been almost unthinkable at the beginning of the century, present-day progressive political leaders like Bernie Sanders and Alexandria Ocasio-Cortez carry the mantle of Occupy's outward-turning desire to serve the beaten-down, atomized 99%. As Dean observes, Sanders' approach to building meaningful solidarity is a genuine coup against America's moribund, oligarchical two-party consensus, which seems to exist only to serve the privileged 1%:

> The left must respond by building solidarity. Taking the side of the oppressed means that we have to make sure the struggles of the oppressed appear as a side, a side in the class war that cuts through them all. We do this by pushing forward . . . Bernie Sanders' slogan, "Not me, us."
>
> ("Not Us, Me")

By the same token, Dene political scholar Glen Coulthard points to the North American Idle No More movement's provenance out of the Occupy moment. As a vibrant locus of solidarity against the colonial politics of recognition, Idle No More has gathered steam out of a powerful desire to assert Indigenous sovereignty, combat environmental degradation and poverty, and form meaningful alliances across previously siloed communities. Drawing on the psychoanalytic anticolonial scholarship and political dissidence of Frantz Fanon,[6] Coulthard insists that Idle No More is, among other things, an intervention on popular liberal representations of forceful dissent as counterproductively reactive and egregiously violent: "forms of Indigenous resistance, such as blockading and other explicitly disruptive oppositional practices, are indeed *reactive* in the ways that some have critiqued" (Coulthard 169), writes Coulthard. He insists that they are nonetheless integral:

> Through these actions we physically say "no" to the degradation of our communities and to exploitation of the lands upon which we depend. But they also have ingrained within them a resounding "yes": they are the affirmative *enactment* of another modality of being, a different way of relating to and with the world.
>
> (Coulthard 169)

In so doing, "they become a *way of life*, another form of *community*" (Coulthard 169).

Animated by the affirmative, communal spirit of a desire for a better, more just world, Idle No More models a form of revolutionary action that metabolizes and redirects the systemic violence of an oppressive corporate-state apparatus. This thriving movement does so not to assume the position of master, garner recognition, or precipitate chaos but rather to rally solidarity, compassion, perspective, and bravery into a hitherto unthinkable "form of community." The ongoing successes of Idle No

More, and other movements like it, suggest that the best response to contemporary modes of hegemony does not reside in the lures of cathartic counterviolence or the seductions of new age panaceas. Only through the difficult, tenuous work of fostering emancipatory community can otherwise atomized individuals hope to engender another modality of being, another way of life.

Notes

1 See Jacques Lacan's *Seminar VII: The Ethics of Psychoanalysis* for a far-reaching examination of the murky relationship between ethics, the demand for happiness, and psychoanalysis. While Aristotle's *Nichomachean Ethics* and *Rhetoric* align the prospect of happiness (*eudaimonia*) relatively unproblematically with the ethical Good Life, Lacan views the contemporary promise of such harmonization as "a form of fraud." There is no good reason, he continues, why psychoanalysts should strive to make themselves "the guarantors of the bourgeois dream" (*Ethics* 303).

2 See Anna Freud's *The Ego and the Mechanisms of Defence*. London: Hogarth Press, 1937.

3 As though in direct conversation with *Fight Club*, Peter Sloterdijk describes the contemporary metropolitan apartment as an "ego cell," a "container for the self-relationships of the inhabitant" (Sloterdijk 537), who employs its medial and architectural affordances to insulate himself from the physical, scopic, acoustic, and olfactory intrusions of overproximal neighbours.

4 In *The Century*, Alain Badiou looks back on the twentieth century and claims that the defining form of political subjectivity of the era was a "passion for the Real," a voracious appetite for the new expressed through the vehement pursuit of "what is immediately practicable, here and now" (56). Those animated by this purifying passion struggle to shatter the deadlocks of moribund bureaucracies and stale conventions by investing their energies in violent breaks imbued with the false promise of authentic immediacy.

5 See Dana Schwarz's article, "Why Trump Supporters Love Calling People Snowflakes." GQ, 1 Feb. 2017, www.gq.com/story/why-trump-supporters-love-calling-people-snowflakes.

6 Fanon, whose political views were profoundly influenced by Lacanian psychoanalysis, proffers his own philosophical-psychoanalytic account of violence in books like *Wretched of the Earth*. See Derek Hook's "Fanon via Lacan, or: Decolonization by Psychoanalytic Means . . . ?" *Journal of the British Society for Phenomenology*, vol. 51, no. 4, pp. 305–319.

Works Cited

Angel, Christina. "'This Theatre of Mass Destruction': Medieval Morality and Jacobean Convention in Palahniuk's Novels." *Reading Chuck Palahniuk: American Monsters and Literary Mayhem*. Eds. Cynthia Kuhn and Lance Rubin. New York: Routledge, 2009, pp. 49–61.

Badiou, Alain. *The Century*. Trans. Alberto Toscano. Cambridge: Polity, 2007.

Burgess, Olivia. "Revolutionary Bodies in Chuck Palahniuk's *Fight Club*." *Utopian Studies*, vol. 23, no. 1, 2012, pp. 263–280.

Coulthard, Glen S. *Red Skin, White Masks: Rejecting the Colonial Politics of Recognition*. Minneapolis: University of Minnesota Press, 2014.

Dean, Jodi. Interview by Joseph G. Ramsey. "Admitting the Communist Desire." *Counterpunch*, 11 July 2013. www.counterpunch.org/2013/07/11/admitting-the-communist-desire.

Dean, Jodi. "Not Us, Me." 26 November 2016. www.versobooks.com/blogs/2970-not-us-me.

Deleuze, Gilles. "Postscript on Control Societies." *Negotiations*. Trans. Martin Joughin. New York: Columbia UP, 1995, pp. 17–82.

Diken, Bülent, and Carsten Bagge Laustsen. "Enjoy Your Fight! *Fight Club* as a Symptom of the Network Society." *Cultural Values*, vol. 6, no. 4, 2002, pp. 349–367.

Edelman, Lee. *No Future: Queer Theory and the Death Drive*. Durham: Duke UP, 2004.

Evans, Dylan. *An Introductory Dictionary of Lacanian Psychoanalysis*. London: Routledge, 1996.

Friday, Krister. "'A Generation of Men Without History': *Fight Club*, Masculinity, and the Historical Symptom." *Postmodern Culture*, vol. 13, no. 3, 2003, pp. 1–22.

Giles, James R. "Violence, Spaces, and a Fragmenting Consciousness in *Fight Club*." *Chuck Palahniuk: Fight Club, Invisible Monsters, Choke*. Eds. Francisco Collado-Rodriguez. New York: Bloomsbury, 2013, pp. 23–43.

Hook, Derek. "Fanon via Lacan, or: Decolonization by Psychoanalytic Means . . . ?" *Journal of the British Society for Phenomenology*, vol. 51, no. 4, 2020, pp. 305–319.

Kavadlo, Jesse. "With Us or Against Us: Chuck Palahniuk's 9/11." *Reading Chuck Palahniuk: American Monsters and Literary Mayhem*. Eds. Cynthia Kuhn and Lance Rubin. New York: Routledge, 2009, pp. 103–115.

Kuhn, Cynthia G. "I Am Marla's Monstrous Wound: *Fight Club* and the Gothic." *Reading Chuck Palahniuk: American Monsters and Literary Mayhem*. Eds. Cynthia Kuhn and Lance Rubin. New York: Routledge, 2009, pp. 36–48.

Lacan, Jacques. *The Seminar of Jacques Lacan, Book I: Freud's Papers on Technique, 1953–54*. Trans. John Forrester. New York: Norton; Cambridge: Cambridge UP, 1988a.

Lacan, Jacques. *The Seminar of Jacques Lacan, Book II: The Ego in Freud's Theory and in the Techniques of Psychoanalysis, 1954–1955*. Ed. Jacques-Alain Miller. Trans. Sylvana Tomaselli. London: Cambridge UP, 1988b.

Lacan, Jacques. *The Seminar of Jacques Lacan, Book VII: The Ethics of Psychoanalysis, 1959–1960*. Ed. Jacques-Alain Miller. Trans. Dennis Porter. London: Routledge, 1992.

Mathews, Peter. "Diagnosing Chuck Palahniuk's *Fight Club*." *Stirrings Still*, vol. 2, no. 2, 2005, pp. 81–104.

McLuhan, Marshall. *Understanding Media: The Extensions of Man*. Toronto: Signet, 1964.

Mendieta, Eduardo. "The Avatars of Masculinity: How Not to Be a Man." *Chuck Palahniuk: Fight Club, Invisible Monsters, Choke*. New York: Bloomsbury, 2013, pp. 45–60.

Palahniuk, Chuck. *Fight Club*. New York: W.W. Norton, 1996.

Robinson, Sally. *Marked Men: White Masculinity in Crisis*. New York: Columbia UP, 2000.

Schwarz, Dana. "Why Trump Supporters Love Calling People Snowflakes." *GQ*, 1 February 2017. www.gq.com/story/why-trump-supporters-love-calling-people-snowflakes.

Simmons, David, and Nicola Allen. "Reading Chuck Palahniuk's Survivor and *Haunted* as a Critique of 'the Culture Industry'." *Reading Chuck Palahniuk: American Monsters and Literary Mayhem*. Eds. Cynthia Kuhn and Lance Rubin. London: Routledge, 2006, pp. 116–128.

Slade, Andrew. "On Mutilation: The Sublime Body of Chuck Palahniuk's Fiction." *Reading Chuck Palahniuk: American Monsters and Literary Mayhem*. Eds. Cynthia Kuhn and Lance Rubin. New York: Routledge, 2009, pp. 62–72.

Sloterdijk, Peter. *Sphere Volume 3: Foams*. Trans. Wieland Hoban. New York: Semiotext(e), 2016.

Ta, Lynn M. "Hurt So Good: *Fight Club*, Masculine Violence, and the Crisis of Capitalism." *The Journal of American Culture*, vol. 29, no. 3, 2006, pp. 265–277.

Vickroy, Laurie. "Body Contact: Acting Out Is the Best Defense in *Fight Club*." *Chuck Palahniuk: Fight Club, Invisible Monsters, Choke*. New York: Bloomsbury, 2013, pp. 61–75.

Žižek, Slavoj. "The Violence of the Fantasy." *The Communication Review*, vol. 6, no. 3, 2003, pp. 275–287.

Žižek, Slavoj. *Organs Without Bodies: On Deleuze and Consequences*. New York: Routledge, 2004.

Žižek, Slavoj. *The Parallax View*. Cambridge, MA: MIT UP, 2006.

Žižek, Slavoj. *Violence: Six Sideways Reflections*. New York: Picador, 2008.

Chapter 12

Self-Removed

Trauma, Irony and Animals

Bo Earle

If trauma designates an event not of meaning but of meaninglessness, a formal break or tear or gap in a very structure of signification, then representing trauma is a Sisyphean task, both necessary and impossible. *Pace* Camus, whether we imagine Sisyphus as happy or sad, triumphant or tragic, is beside the point: either qualification is dwarfed by and dissolved into the quantitative frequency, or *rhythm*, of Sisyphus's cyclic routine. Communicating trauma is not a matter of representing any discrete object or event, but of rehearsing such unresolvable rhythm itself. In order to read Sisyphus or trauma, we must *ourselves* be happy *not to know* how the story ends, to imagine Sisyphus's fate as radically idiosyncratic, beyond good and evil. To face such a radically uncategorizable fate embarrasses much conventional metaphysics and morality. But thinkers from Lucretius to Hegel to Lacan and Agamben have likewise characterized the antithesis of trauma – the condition of ongoing, purposive life, popularly called "*sustainability*" – in terms of "*symbolic excess*." The practical infrastructure of cultural life is sustained by acts pursuant to values in excess of the value of mere survival, or "bare life." Animals, both in virtue and in spite of conventionally emblematizing mere survival – or of *symbolizing symbolic dearth* – provide a, if not the, crucial index and occasion for such irony and thereby meaning and living generally.

Unspeakable Compassion

A contemporary *locus classicus* of such embarrassed excess is Derrida's reflection, in *The Animal That Therefore I am*, on the peculiar shame he feels exposing his nakedness to his cat. He notices that it's actually a second order or "meta-"shame: not simple or direct shame of his nakedness but rather a distinct shame generated by juxtaposing this first order shame to the cat's lack of shame and unawareness of nakedness. In front of his cat Derrida experiences a "reflected shame," "a shame ashamed of itself" (373). This second order shame seems to reveal for Derrida a second order nakedness as well ("seeing myself seen" [380]): this is the naked need for language, compulsively generating ever more language, expressed even in the very naming

DOI: 10.4324/9781003212072-13

of this naked need as such. The "spectacle" of this compulsion to language feeding off of itself is vertigo-inducing, exposes an "abyss" pulling at him, a pull that's only strengthened by his own figure of the abyss.

This vertiginous second-order shame and nakedness lead Derrida to reflect on the role of animals in the Genesis story of the origin of language and knowledge and time. "God destines the animals to an experience of the power of man, *in order to see* the power of man in action" (386). God would see us seeing animals. As a figure for this second order "seeing seeing," the figure of God promises to contain the abyss, to assure us that it's not an empty, naked compulsion but rather an omnipotent plenitude. But this promise of containment, like any other linguistic figure, just returns to the same vertigo-inducing otherness of the animal:

> God wanted to oversee but also abandon himself to his curiosity, even allow himself to be surprised and outflanked by the radical novelty of what was going to occur, by this . . . event of naming whereby Ish would begin to see them and name them without allowing himself to be seen or named by them. . . . This . . . marks at the same time the infinite right of inspection of an all powerful God *and* the finitude of a God who doesn't know what is going to happen to him with language . . . the finitude of a God who doesn't know what he wants with respect to the animal, that is to say with respect to the life of the living as such.
> (386f)

On the basis of this, what Derrida terms "God's exposure to surprise" (387), Derrida introduces this essay's key pun, turning on the interchangeability, in the first person singular, of the French verbs "to be" and "to follow." Making us hear these two meanings together is Derrida's way of trying to acknowledge and engage the abyss instead of violently suppressing it. To be is to be after the animal. There's a dual meaning in play here, too: to follow means, on the one hand, to pursue the animal for the sake of naming it, laying claim to knowledge and property but, on the other hand, also to succeed it in time, to be predicated upon animals' primal unnamable presence. This duality – separating an animal's name from this particular creature here to which I can only point – is the origin not just of language but of time:

> God lets Ish call the other living things all on his own, give them their names in his own name, these animals that are older and younger than him, these living things that came into the world before him but were named after him, on his initiative. . . . [M]an is in both senses of the word *after* the animal. He follows him. This "after," that determines a sequence, a consequence, or a persecution, is not in time, nor is it temporal; it is the very genesis of time.
> (386)

Derrida's essay was written for a conference on "the autobiographical animal"; correspondingly, its key concern is the question of what it would entail to write oneself as animal, or to write in an animal mode, which I take to mean a mode that engages rather than suppresses the abyss and its vertiginous splintering of meanings (of being into being/following, of following into pursuing/ succeeding). I'd lump what this seems to entail for Derrida under four broad headings:

1. Derrida would liberate autobiography from confession, from the restrictive economy of normative truth:

> Autobiography becomes confession when the discourse on the self does not dissociate truth from an avowal, thus from a fault, an evil, an ill. And first and foremost from a truth that would be due, a debt in truth that needs to be paid off. Why *would one owe* truth?
>
> (390)

Derrida's term for such an animal language – what Bataille termed a "general (as opposed to restricted) economy" of symbolic excess, signification without debt – combines the French terms for "animal" and "word" to produce *animot*. A language unindebted to truth would not privilege speakers over non-speakers:

> The suffix *mot* in *l'animot* should bring us back to the word . . . the nominal language of the word, the voice that names and that names the thing *as such*. It would not be a matter of "giving speech back" to animals but perhaps of acceding to a thinking, however fabulous and chimerical it might be, that thinks the absence of the name and the of the words otherwise, as something other than a privation.
>
> (416)

2. Derrida would mobilize *compassion* as a kind of expressivity in passivity. Thinking the lack of language otherwise than as privation requires "terms . . . to be inverted": requires a "reversal in the essence of nature" (388). "Nature (and animality within it)" (388) is sad, Derrida says, not because it lacks language but because it has been invaded by language:

> the form of the question changes everything. It no longer simply concerns the *logos*, . . . having it or not, nor does it concern more radically . . . this *habitus* that one calls a faculty or "power," that can-have or the power one possesses (as in the power to reason, to speak and everything that that implies). The question is disturbed by a certain *passivity*. It bears witness, manifesting already, as question, the response that testifies to a sufferance, a passion, a not-being-able. The word *can*

> [*pouvoir*] changes sense and sign here once one asks "can they suffer?" The word wavers henceforth . . . "Can they suffer?" amounts to asking "can they *not be able*?" . . . Being able to suffer is no longer a power, it is a possibility without power, a possibility of the impossible. Morality resides there, as the most radical means of thinking the finitude that we share with animals, the mortality that belongs to the very finitude of life, to the experience of compassion, to the possibility of sharing the possibility of this nonpower.
>
> (396)

3. Such an impossibility could only be communicated by a *compulsively irresistible kind of compassion*. If normal meaning and reason depend for their communication on logical norms and mental certainty, compassion is transmitted more like a contagious compulsion. Surrendering to this compulsion is finally what it means to *follow* as a mode of being:

> With this question – "can they suffer?" – we are not standing on the rock of indubitable certainty. . . . But from another perspective we are here putting our trust in an instance that is just as radical, however different it may be, namely what is undeniable. No one can deny the suffering, fear or panic, the terror or fright that humans witness in certain animals. . . . [T]he response to the question "can they suffer?" leaves no doubt. In fact it has never left any room for doubt; that is why the experience we have of it is not even indubitable; it precedes the indubitable, it is older than it. No doubt either, then, for the possibility of giving vent to a surge of compassion, even if it is then misunderstood, repressed, or denied, held in respect. Before the *undeniable* of this response. . . , before this response that precedes all other questions, the problematic changes ground and base.
>
> (396–397)

4. Engaging such compulsive compassion would mean *reconstituting language as animal*. Sustaining this "change of problematic" requires a discourse devoted to transgressing but therefore also fostering limits, making them, as Derrida says above, "waver."

> Whatever I say is designed, certainly not to efface the limit, but to multiply its figures, to complicate, thicken, delinearize, fold, and divide the line precisely by making it increase and multiply.
>
> (398)

> The discussion becomes interesting once, instead of asking whether or not there is a discontinuous limit, one attempts to think what a limit becomes once it is abyssal, once the frontier no longer forms a single

> indivisible line but more than one internally divided line, once, as a result, it can no longer be traced, objectified, or counted as single and indivisible. What are the edges of a limit that grows and multiplies by feeding on an abyss? . . . [A] multiplicity of organizations of relations between living and dead, relations of organization or lack of organization among realms that are more and more difficult to dissociate by means of the figures of the organic and inorganic, of life and/or death. There relations are at once close and abyssal, and they can never be totally objectified. They do not leave room for any simple exteriority of one term with respect to another. It follows from that that one will never have the right to take animals to be the species of a kind that would named the Animal, or animal in general.
>
> (399)

Derrida's concluding rejection of a discourse of rights connects his esoteric ruminations on animals with the work of one of the most familiar and longstanding animal theorists, Peter Singer. Singer questions the discourse of animal rights on the grounds that securing a right that could pertain to both human and non-human animals would incur too much of a cost to the aggregate interest of all animals. In a nutshell, this claim boils down to the trade-off between freedom and equality: Singer says that securing equal rights for all undermines the freedom of each. Animal rights are all about preserving and protecting the principle of the inherent value of the individual. Singer argues against this principle because he contends that individuality per se lacks such value and gains it only through *actual pursuit of particular interests*. Hence, instead of animal rights, Singer advocates utilitarian maximizing of animal interests, "liberating" the contingent interests of individual lives as values to be maximized in aggregate even though this will inevitably entail unequal costs for some individuals.

Tom Regan's complaint against Singer's utilitarian position is that it casts individuals as mere "receptacles" for their interests. While Singer maintains that individuality is not a value in its own right but only in pursuit of certain interests in certain circumstances, he specifies that one such interest consists in the organism's perpetuation of its own life (19). That is, individual interest is not limited just to *getting* satisfaction instead of suffering but is crucially also about *pursuing* preferences regardless whether these are satisfied or not. This is true of non-human as well as human animals: we all have a distinct interest in *the act itself of pursuing* what we want above and beyond the question of whether or not we get it. Due to this distinction, Singer calls himself a preference utilitarian as opposed to a hedonistic utilitarian.

So, Singer doesn't reject the right of individuals to make their own choices; he sees this value not as absolute but as continuous with and relative to the whole array of interests that individuals can have. Singer concludes that any human or non-human would prefer to incur some risk of self-sacrifice for the sake of *having a chance at* maximizing individual interests (20). Whereas animal rights advocates would rather eliminate such risk by equalizing interests (and thereby necessarily homogenizing, de-individuating) them, Singer sees such restrictions as disproportionately undermining pursuit of individual preferences.

Thus, Singer arguably implies that accepting some risk of death is an existential condition of exercising preference. This is consistent with Singer's very prominent utilitarian defense of euthanasia, but it seems significant that here accepting some risk of death emerges not as an incidental cost of maximizing interests but as a condition of the pursuit of animal preference per se. That is, the acceptability of euthanasia for the sake of exercising preference doesn't depend on certain relatively extreme circumstances but is a condition of life as such.

The contention here also arguably could be associated with a Nietzsche's radical fatalism, or pragmatic ontology, according to which a thing *is* what it *does*: lacking the prerogative to act on its own preferences, an organism lacks a proper existence per se. Richard Dawkins's functional, ecological definition of species illustrates this point by demonstrating that no actual organism does not mark its environment, effecting what Dawkins terms an "extended phenotype." To mention only the most obvious example of a principle that applies to all beings: a beaver's phenotype cannot be limited to the beaver's static body, since this body *means nothing* in remove from its actual environmental *functions*, such as dam building. Nothing exists except in the concrete context in which it's effected, where its effects are felt, where it *interacts* or *becomes in interaction with* its irreducibly diverse, ever-changing context. As Dawkins puts it:

> Genes manipulate the world and shape it to assist their replication. It happens that they have "chosen" to do so largely by moulding matter into large multicellular chunks which we call organisms, but this might not have been so. Fundamentally, what is going on is that replicating molecules ensure their survival by means of phynotypic *effects upon the world*. It is only incidentally true that those phenotypic effects happen to be packaged up into units called individual organisms.
>
> (5)

Well before Dawkins, the less-renowned, early 20th century zoologist Adolf Portmann likewise lamented how scientific pursuit of supposedly objective causes leads us to disregard surface effects (204). Specifically, Portman examines the way the kind of extended expression Dawkins describes as serving the affective social bonds evoked by Derrida and Singer. The result for Portmann is a notion of existential or psychological value as inextricable from external display. Portmann describes animal morphology as manifesting "the inner psychical world of the animal" on the surface: bodies develop primarily as means for "transmitting" and "receiving" signals of this psychical world (185). Portmann notes that what is morphologically most superficial is often what's most essentially distinctive of that species (213f).

> The morphological features have a special form value which cannot be understood as a function of preservation or as structures for manifesting changes in mood. This form value makes visible to us the special natures of each particular organism. . . , [its] "displayed existential value" [or] presentation value.
>
> (214)

In other words, what we've been discussing as the kind of symbolic excess that binds human communities together in the name of values above and beyond biological survival, Portmann posits as the aim of animal life as well: "the production of forms of the animal body goes far beyond the elementary needs for preservation" (201) and notably includes, Portmann says, "the semantic or cryptic" (208). The isolated, static animal body (no less than the isolated static human body) becomes merely the interface or medium of this dynamic system of social communication. As in Roughgarden, the overarching evolutionary imperative is just to increase the productivity of communication and collaboration, where productivity is measured by no criterion other than diversification and variegation of the system of communication itself, the enrichment of its concrete effects, what Portmann terms "one of the most universal phenomena of all: the constant production in the course of the earth's history of new variants, of new organic forms, and the incessant alternation of organic life" (203). Hence, Portmann concludes,

> We are not confronted with creatures whose essential nature we shall understand fully. . . . All around us are forms of life, small or large, in which have been realized other possibilities of existence than those found in our own lives. . . . Perhaps this book on animal forms, by presenting some aspects of the problem of shapes as a whole, may serve to remind us that the inwardness, that great mystery of living creatures, speaks to us through these many and varied forms. . . , [and hence that the] understanding . . . must completely permeate a more comprehensive knowledge of the forms themselves, if our relationship to other lives is not to be mere undirected roving of the emotions, but the way to a true and deepened inner experience.
>
> (220f)

"Learning to Listen"

As nomadic buffalo hunters, the Crow developed the practice of "counting coups" as a way of maintaining temporary yet indisputable proprietary claims to hunting territory. According to Jonathan Lear's account in *Radical Hope: Ethics in the Face of Cultural Devastation*, it is precisely the symbolic excess of this practice that creates Crow territory as an indisputable reality. It is remarkable that the term "counting coups" applies equally to the act itself of challenging enemies and subsequent ceremonial honoring of this act: as if accomplishing an heroic deed were on some level one and the same as being honored for such a deed, underscoring the importance of symbolic excess for the construction of cultural reality. The ultimate purpose of the deed is not just to ward off invaders but to perpetuate cultural meaning as an end in itself, to sustain a cultural reality.

> So when the Crow went on the reservation, and gave up nomadic buffalo hunting, they didn't just lose an incidental means of subsistence but the basis upon which their reality and world were structured. Hence Plenty Coups' haunting statement, "after this, nothing happened"; the world of properly Crow experience effectively ended, relegating them to a ghostly afterlife in which they maintained the nominal status of Crow tribesmen without being able to execute the practices of effective Crow subjectivity. "One symptom of this," Lear writes, "is that. . . *a peculiar form of irony will first become possible.* . . . One could now ask: *Among the warriors, is there a warrior? . . . Among the Crow, . . . is there a Crow?*"
>
> (44, 47)

According to Lear, overcoming this collapse of Crow reality, or cultural devastation, requires inventing new ways of insisting on symbolic excess, or in other words "a new Crow poet":

> one who could take up the Crow past and – rather than use it for nostalgia or ersatz mimesis – project it into vibrant new ways for the Crow to live and to be. Here by "poet" I mean the broadest sense of a creative maker of meaningful space. The possibility for such a poet is precisely the possibility for the creation of a new field of possibilities.
>
> (51)

Such a poetry arrives in the form of Plenty Coups's dream of the chickadee. In this dream, Plenty Coups is told to "*become a chickadee!*"

> He is least in strength but strongest of mind among his kind. He is willing to work for wisdom. The Chickadee-person is a good listener. Nothing escapes his ears, which he has sharpened by constant use. Whenever others are talking together of their successes and failures, there you will find the Chickadee-person listening to their words.
>
> (80)

Lear emphasizes the *irreducible ambiguity* of this dream: it provides a resource for dealing with cultural collapse because it suggests a *form* of purposeful practice, and even standards of excellence for performing this practice, without providing specifics, leaving all the practical details to be determined: what it means to be a good listener, strong of mind and wise are all radically open for negotiation, to be decided according to how things play out in a future that is as yet totally unclear.

> There is no first-order advice at all – unless "learning to listen" counts as first-order behavior. Part of what it is to acquire the virtue of the chickadee is to be able to spot what the "successes" and the "wisdom" of others are – and to learn from them. The wisdom of the chickadee consists in being able to recognize the genuine wisdom of others.
>
> (81f)

How one goes about gaining the "wisdom of recognizing wisdom" isn't as clearly mapped out as coup counting, but it nonetheless suggests the kind of symbolic excess ("being least in strength but strongest in mind") upon which a new cultural reality might be grounded. Indeed, the cultural resources offered by the chickadee dream are arguably all the richer precisely because it is *nothing but* symbolic excess. As Lear notes,

> The dream did not even explicitly predict that the Crow will survive. . . . In this way, Plenty Coups can both bear witness to the end of a traditional way of life and commit himself to a good that transcends these finite ethical forms. Precisely because Plenty Coups sees that a traditional way of life is coming to an end, he is in a position to embrace a peculiar form of hopefulness. It is basically the hope for *revival*: for coming back to life in a form that is not yet intelligible.
>
> (95)

To bear witness to such an end of tradition is likewise to acknowledge life's unfathomable potential or what Agamben terms "The Open." What counts in language as "life" does so against the open-ended horizon of the question of what it means to count at all, to ecologically participate or take part in an unfathomable, cosmic whole:

> Only because the animal voice is not truly "empty" . . . , but contains the death of the animal, can human language, articulating and arresting the pure sound of this voice (the vowel) – that is to say, articulating and retain the *voice of death* – become the *voice of consciousness*, meaningful language.
>
> (45)

To bear witness to such an end of tradition is likewise to acknowledge the "dangerous," or "traumatic," kernel of Darwinian theory. What Darwin called adaptive "fitness" is better characterized in terms of the economic notion of "satisficing," in order to foreground what Darwin himself insisted was the radically accidental and provisional status of any instance of adaptive success. Adaptive success on this view replaces the triumphal conception of determinately satisfying certain fitness criteria with the humbler one of contingently, provisionally sufficing to avoid extinction.

Nietzsche's emphasis on style implies that such rhetorical distinctions can determine much of the reality they seem merely to describe. A thing is nothing other than "the sum of its effects," Nietzsche writes in *Ecce Homo*; but this, like all of his later work, emphasizes that everything he writes is *writing*: the effects of all things are ultimately linguistic. Experience is always a matter of reading. Like Nietzsche's notion of "amor fati," the ultimate significance of the term satisficing is to insist insisting on its rhetorical status and concomitant inability to contain the unpredictability of fate. Likewise, a virtue of the biologist Joan Roughgarden's *Evolution's Rainbow* (2013) is its attentiveness to the rhetorical figures by which these issues are framed. Specifically, Roughgarden advocates switching from the trope of "survival of the fittest" to a rather social rubric highlighting the relative productivity of various forms of coordination. This rhetorical shift is not reducible to a theoretical claim so much as it removes an obstacle to ecological thinking: namely, the undue essentializing of the individual who, whether on the level of the gene or the organism, would embody easily fetishized characteristics of normative fitness. Instead of the trope of the fit individual, Roughgarden proposes that of the provisionally productive community as much richer, more nuanced, capacious and finally productive. In fact, Roughgarden does not just propose a new trope but argues that the evolution of human society may result in a wide variety of family arrangements – "monogamy, polyandry, or polygyny" – and even that the wildly unpredictable turbulence of social dynamics makes "the outcome of social evolution . . . as uncertain as where a white-water stream deposits a floating leaf" (177). Her recourse to the leaf metaphor here instructively indicates that it is finally literary invention that stands to sustain our sensitivity to the diversity of potential social forms. If we cannot unambiguously name or display what it is that keeps extinction at bay, we can try to speak in ways that keep us alive to the unpredictable tumult of the floating leaf.

Consequently, the communal productivity described by Roughgarden paradoxically must involve a great deal of what cannot but appear as unproductive, unaccountable expenditure. Mauss's account of the gift describes the role of waste in what George Bataille termed a "general" as opposed to "restricted economy."

> Economic science merely generalizes the isolated situation; it restricts its object to operations carried out with a view to a limited end, that of

> economic man. It does not take into consideration a play of energy that no particular end limits: the play of living matter in general, involved in the movement of light of which it is the result. On the surface of the globe, for living matter in general, energy is always in excess; the question is always posed in terms of extravagance. The choice is limited to how the wealth is to be squandered.
>
> (Bataille 1991, 23)

Like Roughgarden's productive collective of indeterminately other-than-fit individuals, the gift economy requires participants to divest from the calculus of possessive individuality. Michel Serres suggests that his book *The Parasite* has a millennial mission based in the paradoxically positive enactment of such divestment: to reverse the world order, allowing a primeval gift economy to return and supplant the current economy of restrictive meaning and debt.

> The world turns in one direction; history has its economy where exchange is fundamental: it is called the meaning of history. It stops a moment, turns in the other direction, and in this new story, exchange appears after everything was freely given. It is not a new story; on the contrary, it is an ancient one, lost in the dark recesses of memory. . . . There are only barely perceptible traces of the history of giving in texts and on monuments. Since then, we have been caught up in economic history, a time of calculation and exchanges and of making up for losses. Does this history have an outside? That is precisely the subject of this book.
>
> (30–31)

Serres represents the parasite not just as the trace of a lost and perhaps future gift economy but also and concomitantly as a rhetorical figure uniquely adapted to acknowledging what Roughgarden calls the tumult of social dynamics. In both English and French, the term can serve as a metaphor of itself: if its primary meaning is that of a biological parasite, in both cases its secondary meaning applies this by analogy to the notion of a social freeloader. In French, the term has a unique third signification: "noise," or what surrounds and obscures the signal, which describes the kinds of contingencies that analogical transfers of meaning (for instance from biological to social parasites) elide but also presuppose. In his account of the fable of the city mouse and the country mouse, Serres makes much of the reversibility of the roles of guest and host: the roles are structural and provisional and the individuals who fill them arbitrary. The fable recounts how the city mouse plays guest to a man but host to the country mouse. It is the crucial role of the third term, noise, to disrupt the role players and reveal the provisionality and arbitrariness of their roles.

So, when the country mouse's enjoyment of his host's hospitality is interrupted by the man's noise, the country mouse becomes a kind of host to that visitation. The man is accommodated by the country mouse without knowing it; he receives a hospitality of which he is oblivious, which, according to the logic of the gift, makes it all the more generous. Like a gift economy, the parasite economy is predicated on overabundance. What circulates across this economy are not credits and debts in a stable currency akin to a standard of fitness but ever-new means of figuring excess, communicating what according to any stable norm must appear as indifferently illicit, wasteful or otherwise unfit.

> One parasite chases another out. One parasite (noise), in the sense that information theory uses the word, chases another, in the anthropological sense. Communication theory is in charge of the system; it can break it down or let it function, depending on the signal. A parasite, physical, acoustic, informational, belonging to order and disorder, [is] a new voice, an important one, in the contrapuntal matrix.
>
> (6)

Like the leaf in tumult, the parasite describes the merest form itself of subsisting – or communicating import – on the brink of chaos. Serres casts such subsistence less in terms of an abiding identity than of a paradoxical double negative: a defiance of disintegration, holding noise at bay just long enough to grasp it as noise rather than being consumed by it. In Agamben's words, "human consciousness keeps in itself this animal that still remembers itself 'as removed'" (7). It is because the leaf is radically exposed to the tumult that it can figure tumult as such, just as in Ammons's "Small Song":

> The reed gives way to the wind
>   and gives the wind away.
>
> (1970, 47)

Like the floating leaf, the parasite is a figure of an act of figuration whose self-referentiality, like Nietzsche's, is radicalized to the point of self-generation, the act by which a community pragmatically constitutes itself as a group of participants in such acts, as transmitters and receivers of signals of this sort. Terms like noise, contingency and chaos are finally no less figurative than terms like parasite, tumult and wind. What counts is the two-part act of, in Ammons's terms, giving way: submitting to disruption in order for that disruption then to be grasped as such. The individual voice is sacrificed to recover an impersonal grammar of communication per se. To give the wind away means, on one hand, to cede, to forfeit the wind as something nameable or otherwise containable, to submit to the sovereignty of noise. On the other hand, this is to give the wind a way, a means of effecting itself as such, a way of being not sheer tumult but specifically wind, of containing tumult in a name. Blowing a reed over gives the wind a way to be wind, just as it gives the wind away as "wind," betrays its rhetorical status: not tumult itself but what language salvaged from its effects. The wind is engendered and betrayed at one stroke; the parasitic power of Ammons's poem is to make the act of figuration just barely register on this side of sheer tumult.

Likewise, for Serres, the general economy of the gift can be approached only from within the restrictive economy of debt; noise may be engaged only by way of what Serres describes as a cascade of disruptions that at any moment can appear to flow in but one direction.

> A human group is organized with one-way relations, where one eats the other and where the second cannot benefit at all from the first. . . . The flow goes one way, never the other. I call this semiconduction, this valve, this single arrow, this relation without a reversal of direction, "parasitic."
>
> (5)

"The chain of parasitism is a simple relation of order, irreversible like the flow of the river" (182). Serres's simile here recalls Roughgarden's of the floating leaf but turns the figure in a way that would seem to contradict her insistence on the unpredictability of evolution, implying that, regardless of how tumultuous, the river must ultimately carry the leaf "one-way," downstream. Serres's figure of the arrow in particular seems to underscore his commitment to approaching the parasite from within the same restrictive economy – the world of possessive, predatory, patriarchal individuals – that the parasite stands to dismantle. It is only in the context of normative demand for fitness, progress or ascent that the generous excess of unfitness may manifest as such. This is a key principle of the project of John Keats, whose poetics of waste would make a cultural currency out of the experience of cultural failure, of pursuing and falling afoul of legitimate currencies of cultural prestige.

By way of illustration, I will finally consider one of the sonnets Keats wrote after viewing the marbles Lord Elgin imported to Britain from Greece by sea. Keats's second Elgin marbles sonnet begins just like the first and in the classic manner of his odes, by professing that he is not up to the task:

> My spirit is too weak – mortality
> Weighs heavily on me like unwilling sleep,
> And each imagin'd pinnacle and steep
> Of godlike hardship, tells me I must die
> Like a sick Eagle looking at the sky.
>
> (2001, 291)

Keats invokes an eagle, not to contrast himself with its strength but to identify with its illness. This mobilizes Keats's key trope of non-translatability and his tendency generally to collapse narrative resolution and metaphoric containment into metonymic series and patterns: "curbing magnanimity," as he advised Shelley by letter, and instead "loading every rift with ore" (August 16, 1820, 509). The image of the sick eagle gives us not just non-translatable modes of perception but also a self no longer conversant with its environment. The bird has become a stranger to the element of its existence, the image stretching readers' thought and empathy (our means of deciphering each other and the world) impossibly far. Like Serres, Keats opens up Wordsworth's signature experience of being "admonished from another world" (Wordsworth 1888, VII, 649) by showing that this experience consists essentially in reproduction of images of itself. In the first Elgin marbles poem, Keats calls himself freakishly meek; in the second, this unfitness is made expressive, allegorizing itself first as a body weighted by sleep and next by the sick eagle. The subsequent sestet does not resolve this unfitness but proliferates its allegorization:

> Yet 'tis a gentle luxury to weep
> That I have not the cloudy winds to keep,
> Fresh for the opening of the morning's eye.
> Such dim-conceived glories of the brain
> Bring round the heart an undescribable feud;
> So do these wonders a most dizzy pain,
> That mingles Grecian grandeur with the rude
> Wasting of old Time – with a billowy main –
> A sun – a shadow of a magnitude.
>
> (2001, 291)

Keats juxtaposes legitimate grandeur to its rude wasting, immaculate glory to the vulgar brain, wonder to pain, the sun to the chaos of the wind and sea, the magnitude to its shadow. More important than these juxtapositions themselves is the aesthetic pattern that Keats uses to set them in motion. In fact, these glories are not actual glories but rather "dim-conceived glories of the brain," implicitly illegitimate excretions of a material organ akin to the orphaned tear, the body of a bird too sick to fly and ultimately the billowy main itself, the unfathomable sea of historical fate. Like his "Ode to Psyche," the sonnet finds a new fetish to worship in historical refuse, relishes his tears for their perversely potent symbolism, incarnating bodily excess and liability and accidental historical fate generally. Instead of proper mourning, Keats invokes bereavement in an overtly formulaic way that foregoes determining what is lost. Bereavement here does not turn inward, as in Wordsworth, to reconsolidate the self but explodes the self into open-ended series of self-wasting images of waste. In Keats's sonnet, glories cannot be wasted because they are already waste. As in Ammons, giving way to despair also gives despair a way. The impossible attempt to allegorize despair is integral to the experience of despair as such; there is no despair without it, no despair that is graspable on this side of unfathomable tumult. To communicate despair is to communicate this impossibility, to make ever-new gifts of our endless unfitness.

Works Cited

Agamben, Giorgio. 2003. *The Open: Man and Animal.* Translated by Kevin Attell. Stanford: Stanford UP.

Ammons, A.R. 1970. *Uplands.* New York: Norton.

Bataille, Georges. 1991. *The Accursed Share.* Vol. 1. Translated by Robert Hurley. New York: Zone.

Camus, Albert. 2018. *The Myth of Sisyphus.* New York: Vintage.

Darwin, Charles. 2003. *The Origin of Species.* New York: Signet.

Dawkins, Richard. *The Extended Phenotype.* New York: Oxford UP.

Derrida, Jacques. 2008. *The Animal That Therefore I Am.* Translated by David Wills. New York: Fordham University Press.

Hegel, G.W.F. 1977. *The Phenomenology of Spirit.* Translated by A.V. Miller. Oxford: Clarendon Press.

Keats, John. 2001. *The Complete Poetry and Selected Letters of John Keats.* New York: Modern Library.

Lear, Jonathan. 2008. *Radical Hope.* Cambridge: Harvard UP.

Nietzsche, Friedrich. 1974. *The Gay Science.* Translated by Walter Kaufman. New York: Vintage.

Nietzsche, Friedrich. 2009. *Ecce Homo.* New York: Oxford UP.

Portmann, Adolf. 1967. *Animal Forms and Patterns.* New York: Schocken.

Roughgarden, Joan. 2013. *Evolution's Rainbow.* Berkeley: University of California Press.

Serres, Michel. 2007. *The Parasite.* Translated by Lawrence Schehr. Minneapolis: University of Minnesota Press.

Singer, Peter. 1987. "Animal Liberation or Animal Rights?" *The Monist*, Vol. 70, No. 1, pp. 3–14.

Wordsworth, William. 1888. *The Complete Poetical Works of William Wordsworth.* London: Macmillan.

Index

9781032079134